At the He D1357947
of Alzheimer's

A Complete Guidebook to
Understanding and Caring for a Person
with Alzheimer's Disease

Understanding Alzheimer's Disease

Effective Ways to Handle Challenging Behaviors

Good Communication Techniques • Caregiver Survival Tips

Handling Family Dynamics • Finding Support Systems

Choosing the Best Residential Care Facility

Forging a Partnership for Care

by Carol Simpson

Foreword by Philip D. Sloane, MD, MPH

$\mathcal{F}$OREWORD

❧

As we approach the 21st Century, Alzheimer's disease looms as the largest health problem facing this nation's elderly. A poorly understood disease – which, in fact, is probably several diseases – Alzheimer's disease gradually steals its victims' mental and physical abilities. The disease can last more than a decade, and as a result has a significant impact on families.

Alzheimer's disease always has more than one victim, for those who love the person with the disease suffer tremendously. Not only do they lose a companion, friend, spouse and/or close relative, but they are thrust into the role of being a 24-hour caregiver. The disease, by gradually taking away the mind and personality of the sufferer, leads to behaviors that can be extremely difficult to manage and frustrating for family members and other caregivers.

This guidebook provides two kinds of valuable information for caregivers – reassurance that they are not alone and practical advice on how to manage. The testimonials by well-known personalities are fascinating. The reader both learns from and empathizes with celebrities like Jack Lemmon, Nils Lofgren and Shelley Fabares as they relate their struggles with understanding and managing a loved one with Alzheimer's. The informational material is succinct, concise, and practical.

Until we find a cure for the disease – which seems far off – caregivers need sources of inspiration and information. *At the Heart of Alzheimer's* provides an excellent source.

Philip D. Sloane, MD, MPH

$\mathcal{A}$CKNOWLEDGEMENTS

✺

Making this book a reality was the result of hard work and dedication by many enthusiastic participants.

Without the wonderful people whose stories are quoted throughout the following pages, and their willingness to share the details of their personal lives, *At the Heart of Alzheimer's* would be a hollow shell. Heartfelt thanks go to all the ManorCare Health Services residents and their families who generously gave of their time and insights. Special appreciation is due to Alan Thicke and Nils Lofgren, who helped shed light on Alzheimer's caregiving by sharing their family stories.

I also want to thank wholeheartedly the Alzheimer's disease experts who added so much to the book's content. Philip D. Sloane, MD, MPH, Professor of Family Medicine, University of North Carolina School of Medicine, was instrumental in ensuring the medical integrity of the information herein. Dr. Sloane's extensive experience in caring for individuals with dementia, and his knowledge of current research, assessment and care techniques, lent invaluable insight into these pages.

Lisa Gwyther, MSW, founder and Director of the Duke University Center for Aging's Alzheimer's Family Support Program, also provided a wealth of information on the issues families face when caring for someone with Alzheimer's disease or a related disorder. Ms. Gwyther's willingness to share her tremendous knowledge and insight gives readers fresh perspective and hope.

Also immeasurably adding to the success of *At the Heart of Alzheimer's* were Merle Wexler, Director, Arden Courts Alzheimer's Assisted Living, in Potomac, Maryland, and Anna Marie Landbo, Activities Director, ManorCare Health Services in Elk Grove Village, Illinois.

Last, but certainly not least, I want to thank my coauthor, Kalia Doner. Ms. Doner is Senior Editor at *Working Mother* magazine and author of 17 other nonfiction books on a variety of topics.

CONTENTS

Preface

"When it comes to taking care of a person with Alzheimer's,
you want to know as much as possible about the
disease and how the experts have learned to manage it.
Luckily, there's been a lot of progress in the
past decade in understanding what is best for
the person with Alzheimer's… and for the caregiver.
If you apply these insights,
you'll see positive results."

⌐

Carol Simpson

At the Heart of Alzheimer's is your guidebook to caring for your relative with Alzheimer's disease. It shows you how to efficiently handle whatever situations arise with creativity and flexibility. The key is to think with your head and your heart.

This book is designed to answer your questions and ease your worries about taking care of a relative with Alzheimer's disease. It will provide you with the basic knowledge you'll need to think creatively about handling the demands of your unique caregiving situation. It will also assist you in taking advantage of the many resources available to help you and your relative manage the stresses of living with Alzheimer's disease. And most important, it will show you that as a caregiver you are not alone.

WITH YOUR HEAD

You want to try to remain as objective as possible about your role as a caregiver. Both you and your relative with Alzheimer's will do best if you think clearly about planning day-to-day and long-term care. Try to develop a caregiving plan early in the process. That way you can anticipate and plan ahead rather than react in a crisis situation. The practical advice in this book is designed to help you do just that. You'll:

- become familiar with the latest scientific knowledge about Alzheimer's disease;

- find out how to establish caregiving goals that provide the most supportive environment for the person with Alzheimer's;

- discover effective ways to manage many difficult behaviors;

- learn how to make the house a safe and secure environment;

- develop ways to protect yourself from "caregiver burnout";

- forge workable solutions to family conflicts about providing care for your relative with Alzheimer's;

- find out about professional help that's available for home-based care;

- receive guidance on tackling the difficult decision to move your loved one into residential care;

- learn about the alternatives available if you decide to move your relative into a residential care facility;

- learn how to make the move to a residential care facility as simple and easy as possible;

- establish your continuing role as a caregiver after your relative moves out of the house.

WITH YOUR HEART

Practicality alone won't solve the problems of providing care. It must be joined with emotional involvement if you are going to nurture your creativity, flexibility and sense of humor. These three, all-important qualities will enable you to appreciate the many moments of laughter, joy, admiration, awe and satisfaction that arise during the challenging process of providing care.

By combining a practical outlook with emotional caring, you'll be able to adopt a can-do attitude.

What can I do? What can my loved one do? Then, when unexpected or unusual behaviors arise, you'll be ready to ask yourself, "What will work in this situation?"

If your relative decides it's time to "go to the office," you'll be able to create an instant workplace on the dining room table. You'll find household tasks that satisfy the urge to be productive and busy.

If your mother is determined to repot all your houseplants, you'll be able to think of ways to distract her so she doesn't inadvertently harm your favorite African violets.

When you need help from friends and family, you'll know how to ask and how to gain their support and cooperation.

TIP

Textbook knowledge is invaluable in understanding the disease, but there are no hard and fast rules about responding to the needs of someone with Alzheimer's. Not everyone progresses on the same timetable, and behavior problems are highly individual. You have to think creatively and be flexible in your reactions if you are to provide appropriate, quality care.

For the new caregiver, this book is meant to assist at every stage of caregiving. You may want to read it all at once, or refer to specific sections as the need arises. But either way, we hope you will keep it near at hand as your role of caregiver evolves.

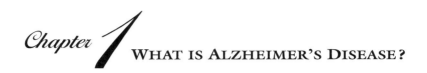

Chapter 1 WHAT IS ALZHEIMER'S DISEASE?

" I always say, when you've met one person with Alzheimer's,

you've met one person with Alzheimer's."

~

Lisa Gwyther, MSW,

Director of the Family Support Program

at the Duke Center for Aging

Alzheimer's is a form of dementia that causes a slow, irreversible degeneration of mental, emotional and physical abilities. There are several types of dementia, but Alzheimer's is by far the most common. The risk of Alzheimer's increases with age — most people are diagnosed in their seventies. But at whatever age it occurs, over time, Alzheimer's makes it impossible to fulfill the demands of independent living.

THE BASIC FACTS

Disruption of a person's mental capabilities usually occurs in adults as a result of delirium or dementia. Delirium is a temporary, reversible condition that may be caused by medication, dehydration, depression, high blood pressure, even thyroid disease. That's why, at the first signs of impaired capacities, a physician should do a thorough evaluation to determine if there is a remedy that will lift the confusion and restore mental functions. If delirium is ruled out, then the cause of mental decline is probably dementia.

Dementia causes the loss of intellectual abilities, which in turn leads to physical incapacities. That process is joined with at least one of the following problems: impaired abstract thinking; disturbance of higher brain functions, such as the ability to name objects; or personality changes. *Alzheimer's disease accounts for 50 to 60 percent of the cases of dementia.* Multi-infarct dementia — small strokes in the brain — accounts for 20 to 30 percent. Between five and 25 percent are a combination of multi-infarct dementia and

Alzheimer's and five percent of cases come from other causes. It is not always easy for doctors to differentiate between these forms of dementia — the best centers are able to diagnose Alzheimer's accurately about 80 percent of the time — but the challenges facing people with all types of irreversible dementia and their caregivers are very similar.

So no matter what the diagnosis, this book offers concrete help for you, the caregiver.

POSSIBLE CAUSES OF ALZHEIMER'S DISEASE

Nerve cell degeneration in the brain seems to be the immediate cause of Alzheimer's. This degeneration is associated with an accumulation of tangled fibers and/or plaques around nerves in the brain — but whether these result from or cause the nerve cell degeneration is not known. In fact, researchers are still searching for an explanation for the changes in mental, physical and emotional capabilities that accompany Alzheimer's disease.

There are several theories. Some researchers believe that Alzheimer's may be related to disruption of acetylcholine, a brain chemical that helps shuttle information across nerve synapses. Another idea is that Alzheimer's is an autoimmune

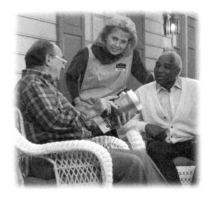

disease in which the body turns on its own healthy cells in the brain. Head injuries are also seen as possible precursors for development of the disease, as are genetic triggers. (However, genes may be the *sole* cause in only five percent of cases.) The newest insights point to changes in brain proteins that may make it impossible for nerves to transmit information.

The most likely scenario, however, is that there is no one cause of Alzheimer's. A person may have to experience multiple triggers to develop the disease. For example, genetic predisposition may make some people more susceptible to Alzheimer's if they also experience a head injury. Untangling the causes and finding a cure remain elusive.

THE SYMPTOMS OF ALZHEIMER'S DISEASE

"Not every person will react the same to Alzheimer's or follow the same timetable," explains Philip D. Sloane, MD, MPH, Professor of Family Medicine, University of North Carolina School of Medicine, "but the symptoms of Alzheimer's are well known."

Over the course of the disease, people with Alzheimer's will develop:

- short-term memory loss, which is often the first sign;

- trouble adjusting to new places;

- confusion about where they are;

- various personality and emotional changes;

- faulty judgment and decision-making abilities;

- trouble expressing thoughts and eventual loss of ability to speak;

- aimless wandering;

- repetitive and erratic behaviors;

- anger and resistance to caregivers.

All Alzheimer's patients show some degree of confusion. Around 60 percent develop minor behavioral problems such as constant requests for attention, suspiciousness and wandering. Less than a quarter demonstrate behavior that is extremely aggressive or socially unacceptable, such as fighting, screaming or making inappropriate sexual advances. Whatever the behavior pattern, people with Alzheimer's gradually lose the ability to perform everyday activities such as getting dressed or going to the bathroom. As the disease progresses, they may become unable to eat or move independently.

As a caregiver, you may be frustrated by the fact that researchers have not discovered the causes of Alzheimer's or a cure for it, but the news is not all negative.

You can take heart in the fact that we've learned how to provide better care for people with Alzheimer's and how to help those who are caregivers. We know what it takes to provide quality care — love, understanding and knowledge. These qualities will allow you as a caregiver to respond to the ever-changing demands of the disease, confident that you have done your best. The best care requires approaches and goals that change depending on the stage of the disease. The love and understanding of thousands of professionals dedicated to providing quality care is also available to you — through many public and private organizations. Together, we can make each day the best that it can be.

THE STAGES OF ALZHEIMER'S

Although not everyone experiences the same symptoms in the same order or with the same time schedule, we can generally characterize the progress of the disease in six stages, which may last three to 20 years. Note that these represent stages of brain deterioration; they can be caused by diseases other than Alzheimer's.

FORGETFULNESS[1]

Very mild cognitive decline:

For example, problems such as: subjective complaints about memory deficit such as placement of familiar objects, forgetting names once known well. There is no objective evidence of deficits in social or employment situations. Don't assume that all confusion and memory loss signal Alzheimer's. Reactions to medications can cause reversible delirium and other medical problems may cause dementia. If you are worried, get a medical diagnosis.

CONFUSION

Early stage: Mild cognitive decline:

For example, problems such as: getting lost when traveling to a familiar location; noticeably lowered performance level at work; trouble finding words and names; little retention from reading; little or no ability to remember names of new people; loss of a valued object; and trouble concentrating.

Late stage: Moderate cognitive decline:

For example, problems such as: decreased knowledge of current and recent events; deficit in memory of personal history; decreased ability to handle travel or finances; and inability to perform complex tasks. Appropriate responsiveness to outside stimulation decreases sharply. Denial of any problem, and withdrawal from challenging situations are common.

DEMENTIA

Early stage: Moderately severe decline:

For example, the person can no longer survive without some assistance. Patients can't remember names of people or places in their lives. They may be disoriented about time and dates. However, they will require no assistance when using the bathroom or eating, but may need help in getting dressed.

Middle stage: Severe cognitive decline:

For example, the person may forget name of spouse and be unaware of events in his or her life. Patients are entirely dependent on others for survival. They may have trouble sleeping in a regular pattern.

Late stage: Very severe cognitive decline:

For example, all verbal abilities are lost and patients need help eating and using the bathroom. Eventually they lose ability to walk; the brain appears to no longer be able to tell the body what to do.

[1]Based on B. Reisberg, Clinical Presentation, Diagnosis, and Symptomatology of Age-Associated Cognitive Decline and Alzheimer's Disease. Alzheimer's Disease: the Standard Reference, New York Free Press, 1983.

Making the Toughest Decision

BY JACK LEMMON

"Alzheimer's is very demanding and frustrating for both the patient and the family. In a world of miracle cures, it is very hard to accept a disease that has no known cause and so far no cure.

"I know the hardships of caring for a loved one with Alzheimer's. Years ago, my wife's mother, whom we absolutely adored, was diagnosed with Alzheimer's, and as it progressed we were faced with having to make some very, very tough decisions.

"The time may come when your family will have to make similar decisions. Some day your loved one may need more care than you can provide at home.

"Making the decision to choose a nursing center is tough. But, by planning ahead before the situation becomes a crisis, by learning about your choices, you'll be able to make the best possible decision for your family."

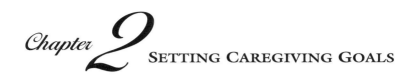

Chapter 2 — SETTING CAREGIVING GOALS

"Sometimes I think that all I need
is for everyone to treat me like a normal person
for just five minutes."

$\backsim$

Gladys R., three years after her
diagnosis with Alzheimer's

*A*ll human hearts long for security, basic comforts, affection and respect. Age and abilities make no difference. Infants who cannot intellectually "understand" their environment react positively to having these needs met, as do people with Alzheimer's who have lost the ability to respond in ways that are familiar to most caregivers. In fact, the challenge to parents of the very young is often similar to that of caregivers of people with Alzheimer's — to understand and fulfill the needs of someone who cannot easily communicate what those needs are.

At times this seems an impossible challenge. It's only normal for frustration to build when it's difficult to decipher the clues. But, caregivers should always remember that what they give makes a difference. The language of the heart can be heard even when there are no words to express it.

THE KEYS TO QUALITY CAREGIVING

As the caregiver, you will find the challenges that lie ahead may be eased if you look for, appreciate and reinforce the mental and physical strengths of your relative with Alzheimer's. You will be well rewarded for the effort — the person with Alzheimer's disease will remain at maximum levels of function, will express less anger and frustration and may have fewer behavior problems. In turn, you will feel less overwhelmed by the caregiving tasks at hand...and in the future.

It's understandable that many families seem to become preoccupied with the deterioration they see instead of taking comfort from and reinforcing what's still positive. However, if you emphasize the strengths, it will help you develop new ways of communicating and interacting effectively. This is not as difficult as it may sound at first. Through most of the course of the disease, a person with Alzheimer's can laugh, communicate, enjoy children, music and pets and remain deeply spiritual.

Jean, who has had Alzheimer's for several years, finds great pleasure in her life, despite difficulty coping with many day-to-day tasks. "My general advice to someone else with Alzheimer's," she says with a smile, "would be to find out what the rules are and be sure to have fun."

Suggested Goals for Caregivers

- Encourage maximum independence and social interaction, while providing security and comfort to the person with Alzheimer's.

- Help your relative with daily personal care activities — but don't do tasks for him or her if they can be done independently. This is important because even though those with Alzheimer's may seem childlike, they are adults and will feel angered or embarrassed if treated like a dependent infant.

- Learn to accept compromise. Allow the person with Alzheimer's to perform tasks and responsibilities in whatever way he or she can, as long as it causes no physical harm or mental anguish — even if the execution doesn't meet your standards.

- Develop new ways of communicating and creative methods of sharing activities. For example, if your grandparent enjoyed going to the symphony, you may not be able to go out to the theater, but you can listen to classical records together at home. Remind yourself of your loved one's previous interests and abilities and encourage him or her to talk about them or help continue to do them.

- Establish a support network — don't isolate yourself. Rely on friends, family and social service organizations to provide day-to-day assistance, counseling and advice.

- Educate yourself about Alzheimer's and its impact on the caregiver and family. The more you understand what is happening to your relative, the easier it is to be patient — and to act appropriately — in the face of often confusing and difficult behaviors.

Creating a Supportive Environment

Often people with Alzheimer's communicate unmet needs in bewildering ways. Frustrated by the inability to tell you what they want, they may wander off, become agitated or argue.

As the disease progresses and new behaviors appear, some will result from changes in the brain and contain little meaning, while others will be increasingly obscure ways of expressing feelings or needs.

The caregiver is constantly faced with the challenge of deciphering and managing these behaviors so that they don't disrupt the household or endanger the person with Alzheimer's — *safety must come first.*

In an attempt to keep the person with Alzheimer's out of harm's way, a caregiver may conclude that restricting the family member's contact with others, limiting physical activity, or removing responsibilities are the most effective solutions. But doing so diminishes the person's quality of life, reduces independence and often causes increased agitation and new behavior problems.

People with Alzheimer's need to remain as physically active and in as much social contact with the world around them as they can comfortably accept. As a caregiver, you want to find ways of managing behavior that allow for freedom and convey respect, lessen the anger and frustration that your

Fire Safety

1. Place smoke alarms throughout the house, including basement and bedroom.
2. Place a fire extinguisher on each floor.
3. Put safety caps over electrical outlets.
4. Keep all matches and lighters out of reach.
5. Use flame-retardant sheets and mattresses.

Preventing Wandering

6. Install child-proof doorknobs or door locks and then camouflage them with curtains or screens that match the color of the door.
7. Install gates across stairways—if the person is unable to climb over them or open them without help.
8. Put electronic buzzers on doors so you know when they've been opened.
9. Lock all windows.
10. Enclose a portion of the yard to provide a secure area for enjoying the outdoors. Remove all poisonous plants, keep garden hoses coiled up, put garden tools out of reach and keep all garden chemicals in a locked cabinet.
11. Lock car keys in a secure place.

Preventing Injuries

12. Secure all rugs with nonstick backings.
13. Keep all hallways clear of furniture and other objects.
14. Put reflector tape on stairs, hallways and bathroom doors.
15. Make sure hallways, stairs and bathrooms are lit at night. Use nonglare bulbs in all areas. During the day let in as much natural light as possible.
16. Avoid highly polished floors.
17. Remove knobs from stove and install safety latches on all kitchen cabinets and drawers.
18. Lock up all alcoholic beverages.
19. Remove lock from bathroom door and make sure medicine cabinet contains no medications, sharp objects or toxic substances. Put all electrical appliances out of reach.
20. Lock up or remove all firearms.
21. Place knives in locked drawers.
22. Unplug microwave ovens.
23. Don't leave hot coffee pots on the counter. Use a thermos to keep coffee warm.
24. Lock away all cleaning products. They can be highly toxic.
25. For your convenience, you may also want to lock the refrigerator so your loved one doesn't overeat or create a mess in the kitchen.

loved one expresses and still protect him or her from harm. There
is a fine balance between protect-
ing someone with Alzheimer's and
restricting that person. While safety
is a key concern, your ultimate goal
as a caregiver is to maximize independence and help the person with
Alzheimer's remain as well-oriented
to the surroundings as possible.
That's why it's so important to
make the environment as safe as
possible. By minimizing danger,
you can allow the freedom your
loved one needs to maintain pride
and self esteem, while maintaining
your peace of mind.

Keeping Your Loved One Active and Involved

Providing a secure environment
will help your relative with
Alzheimer's feel more in control
of his or her life and less angry,
frustrated or afraid. But often
you can do even more to help

ease the difficulty of adjusting to
the disease. When appropriate,
you may include him or her in
decision-making — whether it
involves financial planning or
choosing what clothes to wear.

When a relative is first diagnosed with Alzheimer's, you and
your family may decide he or she
has the mental and emotional
resources to discuss the disease
and make decisions about handling the future. In fact, you may
find that he or she is relieved to
be told about the diagnosis and
welcomes the chance to partake
in decisions about future care
and personal affairs. Often, people will say, "Thank God, you
told me about Alzheimer's. I
thought I was going nuts."

The topics you may want to
discuss are:

• management of financial
  resources;

- establishment of custodianship or conservatorship to allow you oversight of financial resources and authority to arrange for government medical and social benefits;

- assignment of durable power of attorney so a family member can make decisions concerning health care, has full access to health care records and is authorized to hire or dismiss health care providers;

- the writing of a living will to set out instructions for medical intervention in late stages of the disease;

- the writing of a will to resolve inheritance questions;

- establishment of trusts;

- setting up of special bank accounts so that later, when social service agencies need to determine the financial resources of the person with Alzheimer's, there is no confusion about what money belongs to the caregiver and what belongs to the patient;

- how to provide help for the primary caregiver, including schedules for family helpers and the use of outside social services, and choices for nursing home care when needed.

To make such discussions as productive as possible, you and your family may want to consider setting up a series of meetings, instead of trying to settle everything in one intense session. It is also helpful to include objective third parties and expert advisors who can guide the discussion.

- Talking with a social worker, geriatric care manager, attorney and/or clergy may provide you with important information and guidance.

- Asking a medical authority to talk to the whole family about the disease, or attending a workshop, can dispel some misconceptions and outline the medical nature of the disease.

As you and your family develop your caregiving plan, you will find it falls into place more smoothly if you create an environment that balances control and safety with independence and dignity.

BATHING

A person with Alzheimer's should be encouraged to bathe him or herself as long as it is safe. But to avoid falls in the tub, hot-water burns and other hazards, you need to supervise — discreetly at first, and with full participation later as the disease progresses.

Helping your loved one bathe presents several challenges: You may have to deal with his or her anxiety about getting undressed and into the water, being unclothed in front of you or being uncomfortable or confused. You may have to undress the person; you may have to physically support him or her moving in and out of the tub; you may have to wash his or her body. In addition, your loved one may be upset or embarrassed by needing assistance and resist taking a bath.

Sometimes it is useful to give your loved one a sponge bath in bed (slipping a plastic sheet underneath him or her). But when it comes to taking a bath or shower, you are best prepared if you follow the advice that Dr. Sloane offers, based on his extensive research on effective bathing techniques:

- Remember, discomfort or confusion during bathing may trigger fear and agitation. Take time to analyze the person's responses — experiment with eliminating possible sources of discomfort. Be flexible. And if you can't accomplish it today, try a new approach tomorrow.
- Take time to make bathing a relaxing, soothing experience. Never rush or use sudden movements.
- If the person becomes agitated when asked to undress, bathe him or her in the morning before day clothes are put on.
- Try to provide privacy: One method is to allow the person to take his or her clothes off under a large terry towel or cotton sheet and leave it around him or her in the tub or shower.
- To handle agitated behaviors, such as biting and grabbing, try offering distractions and rewards such as food or music. Sing together while bathing.
- If mobility is a problem, provide a seat in the tub or shower for safety and comfort.
- Have the water running and the water and air temperature comfortable before the person enters the bathing area.

TAKING AWAY THE CAR KEYS

Driving is a symbol of independence in our society. For many people it provides an essential link to the outside world. However, as your loved one's ability to reason and make sound judgments decreases, driving can become dangerous. Not only may he or she become lost, responding quickly to a traffic crisis may not be possible and accidents can happen. It is the social responsibility of family and friends to prevent the person with Alzheimer's from injuring him or herself and/or others.

It is always better to be safe than sorry. Many professionals advise families to intervene as soon as the person shows signs of slowing response times, forgetfulness, disorientation and obliviousness to potential danger.

There is no easy way to tell someone that he or she cannot drive any longer. To discuss the driving issue with your loved one you should:

• Speak frankly, but don't be critical. Tell your relative with Alzheimer's that, for his or her own safety, you are going to have to take away the car keys. If the person protests, assure him or her that you understand how difficult it is to accept. Explain that you are doing it for others' safety as well. And make it clear that the decision is nonnegotiable.

• Don't leave car keys out on a hook or in your purse where they are accessible. Keep them with you or find a good hiding place.

• Reassure the person with Alzheimer's that you are available to take him or her wherever he or she wants to go. All your loved one has to do is ask. Explain that you can go for drives or run errands together.

Sometimes the person's doctor can help by discussing the problem with the patient, or, can write a "prescription" to discontinue driving. In difficult cases, a member of the family or the physician can contact the State Motor Vehicle Department for assistance.

It is often a good idea to sell the car of the person with Alzheimer's.

Trial and Error

BY LYNDA O'BRYAN

***Lynda O'Bryan, 33, finds great joy in her
relationship with her grandmother,
who was diagnosed with Alzheimer's 20 years ago.***

"*M*y Nanna lived alone for 11 years after Grandpa died.
Over that time she became more and more forgetful and she
knew it. It made her very isolated because she didn't want to
be around people she didn't feel comfortable with. We had
to stop by her house every day, do her shopping, everything.
But we knew it wasn't a good situation for her. For 10 years
we tried to move her, but she wouldn't budge. Finally, when
she turned 80, we dragged her out of the house. She was
kicking and screaming and grabbing onto the walls. She
wouldn't talk to us. She said she hated our guts. We literally
pulled her out of the house. We had to. She wasn't eating
right. The house was dirty — she had been a spotless house-

keeper. She lived on a very busy road and she couldn't cross the street safely.

"At first we moved her into an independent living situation, in her own one-bedroom apartment — a beautiful facility. She didn't like it. She never settled in comfortably...never developed relationships with anyone there. Even though another resident there stood up at her wedding, that didn't compute. We had to have meals brought up to her room, and she wasn't eating those, either. After a while, we realized that it couldn't go on like that. So Nanna went to live with my aunt and her family for a while.

"After two-and-a-half years they got so burned out. They could never go outside alone. They had to bolt the doors from the inside. The time had come to move her into a nursing home. It was the best thing to do...for everyone.

"The first day we went there she was furious. She yelled, 'I know what you're going to do. You're going to put me in a nursing home and leave me here.' But it turned out to be the smartest place for her to be. She needs a structured set of activities. She calls it 'going to work.' When she went into the nursing home, she was so confused. Now she's more outgoing and 50 percent more with it.

"It's good to keep her busy, even if it's just make-work. Sometimes I'll take all the towels out of the bathroom, mess them up and put them in a basket so she can fold them back up. Or when I go to visit her, if we're not going out, I bring my phone book and we call her relatives to keep connections with people she can't visit a lot. If the conversation is non-sense, it doesn't matter. She likes it.

"We also take her out a lot. We go to church every Sunday and then out to eat with a group of people. She still has command of her social skills to some degree. She was a telephone operator and has always been a good speaker and polite, and that hasn't gone away. So, in public she doesn't say anything inappropriate. For example, she hallucinates, but she won't mention it if there are other people in the car. Then when they get out, she'll ask me, 'Did you see all those ladders or those people dancing in the road?'

"It can be frustrating, though. We take her out and then three hours later she's crying because no one came to visit her. But when she's at church and breakfast, she's enjoying it...then she forgets.

"These days, she forgets more and more. She knows I'm part of the family, but she calls me my mother's name a lot. We go along with it. It doesn't startle me any more. At first it was hard because we were trying to correct her and help her. But we learned that it just makes her angry and frustrated. Trial and error showed us it was better to be flexible.

"The first 10 years are really frustrating; the next 10 years I was getting used to it. But sometimes I wish I could just sit down and talk to her normally. It's sad, although I'm used to it.

"It takes a lot to take care of her and there are people in the family who don't pitch in as much, but it doesn't do any good to fight about it. You just do the best you can. I go there more than my sister because she has such a hard time with seeing Nanna's condition. It's hard on my Mom, too.

"I think one of the most difficult things is that since she got sick, Nanna has become very affectionate. My family's not very expressive or any of that. But when I visit, if Nanna gets tired sometimes we just lie down together and I put my arms around her. She loves it. But my Mom gets uncomfortable.

"None of us could have been prepared for handling Alzheimer's. You have to just try to support each other, even if you can't all contribute the same amount of help. If Alzheimer's teaches us anything, it's not to be too hard on people. Give up a bit of control and just love each other the best you can."

Chapter 3
MANAGING CHALLENGING BEHAVIORS

"Although people with Alzheimer's seldom organize
their environment, they respond to it.
That's why it's important for us to structure the surroundings
to suit individual preferences and abilities."

⌇

Philip D. Sloane, MD, MPH

*F*iguring out how to provide quality care takes time — your solutions will change as the disease progresses. Fortunately, clinical research has developed concrete techniques for coping with behavior problems that will allow you to create a successful, positive environment. By applying these techniques, you will find that you have a great deal of influence and control over how your relative behaves and the quality of life he or she maintains.

BEHAVIOR MODIFICATION TECHNIQUES

Validation, reinforcement, distraction and *alteration of environment* are the most powerful behavior modification tools available to caregivers.

Validation means that as a caregiver you offer support and acceptance for what your loved one believes, even if it may not conform to your concept of reality.

At first, this may seem unnatural or even too accommodating, but the wisdom of the approach is borne out by the results it produces. One woman who struggled daily to cope with the increasingly erratic behavior of her husband, eventually learned that she kept things on an even keel if she just went along with him whenever possible. "I figured out that when he saw a cow in the living room, the best thing for me to do was open the front door and let it out." She validated her husband's perception instead of fighting it, and in exchange he remained calm and did not feel belittled or embarrassed. This example is one of entering into the person's fantasy — an approach of validation.

The key is to remember your goal – to create the most satisfactory relationship possible.

No matter how much you wish that your loved one would just stop "acting crazy" and listen to what you say, people with Alzheimer's cannot change their reality. Challenging can cause your loved one to become agitated and frustrated. Thus, you'll put tremendous stress on yourself and the person with Alzheimer's if you insist that they just "cut it out." Validation allows you to break out of the cycle of negativity by accepting your loved one's point of view, even though you know it may be incorrect or that it may change soon.

Reinforcement means that you provide praise for achievements and good behavior and offer encouragement and guidance as your loved one struggles to attend to life's everyday demands.

"As George began to fade, he could no longer work in the garden," recalls Susan, his wife of 43 years. "He couldn't tell which plants were flowers and which were weeds. One day he dug up all our rose bushes. It made me so angry. I feel guilty now about yelling at him for it, but I couldn't stand the fact that he was incapable." For weeks she kept him out of the garden, fighting with him every time he tried to go out to "work." Then one day she had an idea: She'd create a garden patch in which he could do whatever he wanted. This past summer he joyfully tended to the plot. Susan was able to encourage and praise him, even though his plot was, by conventional standards, a shambles. George's obvious pride and the physical activity helped calm him and give him something to feel good about. Susan was able to stop playing policewoman and to enjoy George's company in the backyard.

You can also practice reinforcement in smaller ways, offering praise for any behavior you want to encourage, and then making sure your loved one has the opportunity to repeat that behavior over and over. For example, if your loved one sets the table for you, offer thanks. Ask him or her to do it for each meal, as long as it provides pleasure. Does it really matter if the knife or fork are in the "wrong" place?

Distraction can be used to deflect your loved one's attention from potential trouble or problem behavior.

One woman reports that her husband, who has been diagnosed with Alzheimer's, still insists on "going to work." When she doesn't let him wander out of the house he becomes angry. But she's discovered that if she breaks into song and starts dancing, he immediately forgets that he wants to "go to work." An enthusiastic ballroom dancer all his life, he is delighted with the opportunity to lead her around the living room in a fox-trot.

Another woman reports that her husband, who is too confused to bathe himself, continually grabs her arm when she attempts to wash him. Finally, she learned to give him a washcloth or a rubber toy to hold. This method of distracting attention can often interrupt the behavior so you don't ever have to speak negatively.

Changing the environment is another useful technique to combat agitation or refusal to cooperate in everyday situations. For example, if your mother becomes upset and refuses to eat when she's seated with the family in the dining room, she may be expressing her discomfort with the situation. Ask yourself questions such as: Is there too much activity or noise? Could she be uncomfortable with having to make so many choices — "Would you like some potatoes?" "Do you want milk to drink?" "Can you pass the meat?"

Such conversation can be quite confusing. To minimize the possible problems, try limiting food choices to only two alternatives, such as "Do you want milk or tea?" Or serve a plate with only one or two foods on it. Try moving her eating area to a quiet spot, away from the TV and the family. Experiment with different chairs to see if she is more comfortable in one than another. Adjust the lighting. It may take time to hit on a combination that works, but you will be able to create at least a temporary improvement.

Altering the environment may also involve changing more personal circumstances. "For about four weeks, my husband was taking his clothes off anywhere, any time. It was so embarrassing. I stopped letting him go outside and was afraid to have anyone visit us," recalls Harriet, who can now laugh at the incident. "I was ready to throw in the towel, until I noticed that he never undressed when he was wearing a certain T-shirt and pants. It turned out that they were loose fitting and 100 percent cotton. Now that's all he wears and he never takes his clothes off in public. He was terribly uncomfortable, but didn't know how to tell me."

As these examples illustrate, caregivers must remain flexible and think creatively. There may be general rules for managing challenging situations, but there are no hard-and-fast solutions.

"Caregivers want to find ways of controlling behavior, but they walk a thin line between accommodating harmless, but uncharacteristic, behavior and preventing their loved ones from harming themselves or others," says Duke's Gwyther.

"It's easy for people with Alzheimer's to feel put down or embarrassed if they are treated like incapable children.

"In the middle stages, they still require outlets for their energy and opportunities to feel productive. While it helps to have routines and structured activities, they want to feel that they are making a contribution and that what they are doing is dignified and meaningful — not just busy work. There is an exception to every rule. That's what makes it so challenging for caregivers."

TIP

It's much easier to change your behavior than to change the behavior of a person with Alzheimer's.

BASIC COMMUNICATION TECHNIQUES

How you communicate with your loved one is as important as what you say. It's easy to lash out in anger or frustration. And it takes time and experience to tailor how you explain things to suit your loved one's level of comprehension.

Camella, who has Alzheimer's and lives in a nursing center in Illinois, is very clear about how she feels people should treat her and others who have memory loss. "I'd tell people to help. Don't say, 'Why did you forget?' Say, 'Let us both go for a walk.' "

The following approaches should make it easier for you to be understood and to get the responses you want.

Get the person's attention. Don't start talking "at" a person with Alzheimer's. Approach quietly, make gentle physical contact by touching the arm or the cheek. Wait until the person is looking at you. Then explain that you want to have a conversation: "I want to tell you something. Can we talk about getting ready to go to bed?"

Eliminate negatives. If you spend all your time saying "no" or "don't," you will upset yourself and you won't get the desired result — a change in behavior. Instead, offer positive alternatives. Rather than saying, "Don't touch the stove," say, "Come look at this beautiful flower." Instead of saying, "Why are you doing that?" distract attention away from the "bad" behavior and rechannel the person's energy into a more positive outlet.

Speak simply and clearly. Short sentences. Repetitive phrases. Basic instructions. And use gestures if words don't seem to get through. All these can help you communicate your desires. If your loved one has trouble eating, don't get into a long, involved discussion. Simply put a bite in your mouth to demonstrate chewing. Then place the food in his or her mouth and say, "Now chew. Okay, now swallow."

Keep your tone warm and empathic. Beware of communicating negative emotions such as anger or disappointment. You don't want to deny your feelings. It's perfectly normal to sometimes feel anger or resentment toward your loved one. But you should try to control when and where you express those emotions. Imposing them on a person with Alzheimer's can cause increased depression in the newly diagnosed and/or agitation in those in more advanced stages of the disease. (For information about caregiver support groups and techniques for easing burnout, see Chapter 6: Professional Help for Home-Based Caregivers.)

Ask simple questions. Limit the number and complexity of decisions you are asking the person to make. Break up involved tasks into simple steps. And wait for responses. Don't become impatient and fill in the blanks or rush ahead to the next set of ideas.

Avoid baby talk. In the early and middle stages of Alzheimer's many people are acutely aware — and sensitive about — failing abilities. Baby talk is embarrassing and insulting. And since people with Alzheimer's may not be able to tell you directly that your manner is upsetting to them, they may become unresponsive, angry or hostile in order to let you know that you are speaking inappropriately.

Remember your loved one's irrational or confusing behavior is a way to communicate feelings or needs. It's not done to irritate you. To probe the meaning of any behavior, ask yourself: What is happening? What could be the cause? Does the behavior express a physical need such as thirst or hunger? Does it express frustration over lack of structure or too much outside stimulation? Then ask, who is involved when the behavior occurs? Where does it occur? When does it occur — around meal times, in the evening? Answers to these questions will help you understand what your loved one is communicating and allow you to make required changes to alter the behavior.

Offer praise and encouragement. Whatever the person does — whether it's going out to dinner with the family, helping you fold the laundry or changing clothes — make sure you say how much you appreciate the help. Encourage positive behavior and you will be more likely to see it repeated.

TIP

To make sense of difficult behaviors, keep a log for a week, recording when and where they occur. Make note of time of day, who's around, other activities that occur at the same time, what the person says or does and how you respond. You'll be surprised at the insights you can gather by looking for patterns.

❈

Managing Specific Behaviors

As the disease progresses, new coping skills are required to provide security and basic comforts. Don't expect to know automatically how to handle new situations. You need to learn to cope with everyday activities, such as eating, bathing or going out. Although you can often rely on your intuition or common sense, there are "tricks" that experts in the field have developed that can help you recognize symptoms of behavior problems, ease the burden — and make both you and your loved one happier and more satisfied with life.

Anger and Agitation

If your loved one becomes angry or agitated for "no apparent reason," you can get agitated yourself. Feeling helpless to identify or correct the behavior takes a great toll on you. But your anger and frustration can simply add fuel to the fire. In such a situation, you want to take a deep breath and step back for a minute. Even in the middle of bewildering confrontations, there are tools you can use to ease the crisis.

First, you may find it helpful to remember two types of triggers for agitation or anger – physical (medical) causes and environmental causes.

Physical causes include trouble sleeping, fatigue from lack of sleep, adverse side effects from medications, failing eyesight or hearing, physical discomfort caused by constipation, pain or fever, or loss of control due to changes in the brain (which may cause hallucinations and paranoia).

Environmental triggers may include too many people or too much activity; sudden or overwhelming noises; unfamiliar places, people or sounds; feelings of abandonment caused when the person with Alzheimer's is left alone or with unfamiliar people; or changes in lighting from light to dark or dark to light.

Task overload happens because people with Alzheimer's can have difficulty handling more than one thing at a time, often do not like changes in daily routines and have trouble coping with fast-paced activities.

Persons with Alzheimer's generally remain highly sensitive to the actions and attitudes of those around them — even if they can't express that sensitivity clearly. They are keenly aware of anger and resentment, and are upset when others argue or are inconsiderate. In fact, according to Dr. Sloane, the greatest success in reducing agitation and frustration happens when caregivers learn to carefully control how they act toward and around the person with Alzheimer's.

To determine possible triggers in your loved one, you must first rule out medical problems and reactions to medications. This medical evaluation should include vision and hearing tests. If you can rule out these causes, move on to eliminate other possible triggers. Provide quiet times at regular intervals, and whenever possible plan activities only when the person is well rested. Provide regular exercise to help release stress and pent-up energy. Make sure the environment is uncluttered and simple, with familiar objects unchanging from day to day.

Experimenting with different approaches can usually reveal ways to ease anger and agitation that work at least some of the time.

It also helps to tell your relative that you understand that he or she is angry or upset by what is happening to him or her. Respect and validation of feelings helps people with Alzheimer's, just as it helps you. It may be okay to let the person know you're sad. That validates his or her perception of the situation.

If all else fails, medications to ease agitation may be needed, but they can cause undesirable side effects — such as sleepiness, movement and walking problems, dry mouth, constipation and bladder problems — and even increased agitation. If behavioral modification techniques don't work, and medication is necessary, stay in close communication with your family member's physician. Sometimes several medications or dosages must be tried before the right treatment is found.

TIP

Alzheimer's can make people behave inconsistently. In the early stages, at one moment they're completely competent, able to play cards or discuss a movie plot, the next they may forget how to get a soda from the refrigerator. They may even be able to function well at work, but be completely confused about how to get from home to the office.

This happens because of the specific areas of their brain that have been affected by the disease. However, for a caregiver, it can be maddening. You may even feel like your loved one should be able to control the confusion, if he or she only wanted to. That's not the case, however. Such behaviors are not intentional, nor are they designed to hurt your feelings.

Wandering

Wandering can be terrifying. One moment your loved one is sitting quietly, the next he or she has slid out the back door and is heading down the street. You can't watch your loved one every moment, but you fear for his or her safety if you don't. Security measures, such as locking the doors, may not work.

There are many possible causes of wandering:

- physical changes in the brain;
- reactions to medication;
- frustration or impatience with what's going on around them or with the activities in which he or she is participating;
- a need to go to the bathroom;
- a desire for exercise;
- a return to the past — so the person thinks it's time to go to work, or to pick the kids up from school;
- physical pain or discomfort;
- hunger or searching for food;

- the idea of going out may be triggered by seeing overcoats, boots or scarves.

Nighttime wandering may involve these triggers. It is also likely that the wanderer can't tell day from night or doesn't expend enough energy during the day to sleep through the night. In some cases, dreams become so vivid that the person can't tell the difference between what is real and what is dreamed.

To lessen the danger of wandering, try:

- making the immediate physical area safe for wandering and then letting the person go;
- providing ample exercise by going for walks around the neighborhood;
- taking a drive;
- labeling rooms, particularly the bathroom, with bright signs incorporating both words and pictures, so that the person can easily find his or her destination in the house;

- reinforcing the concept of time of day, by using large digital clocks that are marked with A.M. and P.M.

Dressing

Being able to dress oneself has enormous impact on self-esteem and dignity. For a person with Alzheimer's, losing this skill can cause depression, anger and confusion. And for the caretaker, it represents one more arena of potential stress. Certain physical changes in motor skills, memory and decision-making abilities can make it unrealistic for many people with Alzheimer's to continue the task unassisted.

There are, however, many "tricks" you can use to make dressing easier. Whatever techniques you use, allow the person to do as much for himself as possible.

"TRICKS" FOR DRESSING

Create a morning routine so the person becomes accustomed to getting dressed after bathing and/or brushing teeth. Don't vary the order.

Reduce or eliminate choices. Hang only one outfit in the closet or no more than two shirts or two dresses so there isn't pressure to make a complex decision. Stick with favorite clothing, buying duplicates if necessary to provide a fresh change of clothes daily.

Label dresser drawers (underwear, shirts, socks) or lay clothing out in the order it is to be put on.

Simplify clothing. Replace snaps, buttons and zippers with Velcro closures. Slip-on shoes with nonskid soles are easy to put on.

Expect the person to handle only one task at a time. It's easy to forget that putting on pants and a belt may need to be broken down into two distinct steps.

Provide step-by-step coaching.

Remember that getting dressed is a personal act that should be done in private whenever possible. It can make some people self-conscious or uncomfortable to get dressed in front of someone else, even a close family member.

Undressing at inappropriate times is the flip side of the problem. When it occurs, look for a reason. Sometimes it expresses discomfort or the need to go to the bathroom. (Watch for tugging or pulling at clothes as a sign.) If you can't figure out the cause, and persuasion fails, try putting clothes on backwards so closings are out of reach. And remember, the person is rarely undressing to be sexually provocative or to cause you embarrassment.

Incontinence

Managing incontinence can be extremely upsetting and logistically difficult. You want to enlist the help of your relative's doctor in finding solutions and exploring possible medical causes, such as a bladder infection or a reaction to medication.

The key to minimizing incontinence is taking the person to the toilet before the bladder empties spontaneously. This can sometimes be accomplished by watching for signs, such as pulling on clothing or touching genitals. Often, a toileting schedule is necessary. Every two hours is an interval that works for many people. Medications can help increase the length of time between episodes of spontaneous urination.

Other possible solutions include:

- eliminating caffeine; it is a diuretic;

- providing liquids on a regular schedule;

- figuring out if there is a pattern to the times wetting occurs and take the person to the bathroom in anticipation of the need;

- toileting before and after eating and right before bedtime;

- making the task easier for your loved one by communicating instructions simply and making sure the bathroom is uncluttered and accessible and toilet paper is in plain view;

- praising the person when he or she uses the bathroom successfully;

- making sure clothing is easy to take off in the bathroom;

- using absorbent pads and/or panties;

- at night, providing sufficient lighting for the person to find the bathroom easily;

- placing a chair-style toilet by the bed.

Remember, many people with Alzheimer's remain acutely aware of their deficiencies. You will embarrass them by criticizing or showing your distaste for the task at hand.

Paranoia and Hallucinations

Sometimes, a person with Alzheimer's may fixate on the idea that he or she is being robbed or conspired against. For example, he or she may develop the habit of hiding valuables or money, forgetting where it is and then accusing a family member of stealing. Or, Alzheimer's can create hallucinations, so your relative may see or hear things that are not there. And, he or she may remember the details of these delusions, but forget events that really happened.

As a caregiver, your patience and understanding may be sorely challenged when a loved one loses touch with apparent reality, especially if he or she begins accusing you of hurtful or deceitful behavior. At such a time, it is vital to remember that the person cannot control these symptoms of the disease. They are not directed personally at anyone. If they don't cause the person with Alzheimer's any harm, it is often best to ignore or accept them.

However, forgetfulness or the idea that someone is "out to get me" can cause the person with Alzheimer's to become over-wrought. When that happens, you want to defuse the situation.

Begin by trying to provide a constant sense of security and routine so the person feels that his or her world is familiar and unthreatening. Instead of removing a valuable so your loved one can't hide it, which may only increase the sense of loss and confusion, try to sleuth out favorite hiding places so you can quickly locate the missing item. Or replace it with a similar object.

Sometimes accusations result from a sense of loss. In that case, offer sympathy. For example, one man found that his father was convinced that he'd stolen his car. He'd tell him over and over, "I did not steal your car. You sold it. How could you think I'd take it?" But his father never absorbed the information and only became more agitated.

After a week of pointless back and forth on the subject, the son realized he was never going to get anywhere until he figured out what triggered the accusation. He asked himself: What is Dad really saying? Why does he keep thinking about the car? When the son remembered how proud his father had been of the car and how trau-matic it had been when they'd had to stop him from driving any more, the son stopped defending himself from the false accusation and instead would say, "I know how much you loved driving around. You miss the car and I do too. Remember when we used to drive out to the beach?

We had so much fun. Would you like to go for a ride in my car now?" This validated his Dad's basic emotion and offered him an avenue for replacing the sorrow with a pleasurable activity.

Other fears may be triggered by confusion over an unidentified noise, such as traffic, or because shadows and dim light make it impossible for the person to make out the surroundings. Many people with Alzheimer's are aware of their vulnerabilities and are afraid that they will not be able to handle threatening or dangerous situations. Shadows and darkness can stimulate these anxieties. In such situations, changes in their brain may cause them to "see" frightening images. Good lighting, which is neither too harsh nor too dim and does not create shadows or glares, and an uncluttered environment may help eliminate such responses.

Occasionally, paranoia and delusions become so overpowering that they are present much of the time. When this happens, everyday events, such as a truck passing in front of the house, can trigger agitation or fear. Or a single false belief may become so intense that it disrupts the household. Medications can often help. Tell your physician what has been happening and work with him or her to find a therapy that controls the paranoia or delusions. Side effects can occur from medications, so notify the doctor if you think your relative is experiencing a negative reaction.

Sexual Misbehavior

Sexual expression is a normal part of life. However, when Alzheimer's disease develops, sexual feelings can lead to actions that are embarrassing to others. These include talking "dirty" or unwanted or inappropriate touching of others or oneself.

Such behavior can be difficult for the caregiver to handle, but you should keep in mind that these behaviors are almost never a threat to others and that the person with Alzheimer's is likely to pass quickly through the stage and leave the behavior behind.

Furthermore, many actions, such as disrobing or inappropriately touching oneself or others, are not meant to be provocative or sexually expressive. Instead, they are an attempt to communicate an unstated need or emotion. Uncomfortable clothing, skin irritation, undiagnosed medical problems such as urinary tract infections or intestinal obstructions, as well as gynecological problems caused by yeast infections or itching that results from lack of estrogen, may cause a person to touch the genital area.

Inappropriate touching of others often represents a desire for contact, a need for reassurance or trouble seeing clearly. Sometimes delusions or hallucinations may be the cause. For example, a woman may be fixated on having nursed her children or thinks that other people are nursing babies.

It is not uncommon for a person with Alzheimer's to mistake someone for a spouse. While this can be upsetting to family members, remember that, again, he or she may crave companionship or human touch. Some wives and husbands report that, although it can be uncomfortable, they are glad their spouses have found friendship and pleasure in another person.

To curb behaviors that make you uncomfortable, you want to figure out the motives:

- Ask your doctor to determine if there are medical problems causing the behavior.
- Try altering the environment to eliminate over-stimulating or agitating noises or activities.
- Make sure clothing is comfortable.
- Rely on distraction to shift attention to other activities.
- Sometimes, providing a back rub, holding hands or rubbing lotion on your loved one's hands and face will provide the soothing touch he or she may be seeking.

A daily log, recording when and around whom such behaviors occur, may also shed light on the triggers and suggest solutions. And always remember, the person is not intentionally trying to be uncooperative or to embarrass you.

Eating

Difficulty with eating is common throughout Alzheimer's disease, especially in the middle and late stages. People with Alzheimer's often lose their desire for food, forget to eat or refuse to eat. For the caregiver this can be frustrating and worrisome. It may even feel like a rejection of care. But rest assured, that is not the motive or cause, and your loved one with Alzheimer's is simply expressing physiological or psychological difficulties through eating behavior.

For you, the caregiver, the important thing is to look for a cause and find a satisfactory solution. Research into management of Alzheimer's-related eating disorders has uncovered some interesting options.

Refusal to eat may be the result of depression over the diagnosis. It may also express a negative reaction to certain flavors or textures of food. Trial and error should help caregivers determine which foods are pleasing and which are not. If the person with Alzheimer's no longer will eat any vegetables, or some other nutritionally important category of food, try changing the texture to something easier to chew and swallow. If necessary, liquid nutritional supplements may be needed to round out the diet. If the person is willing to eat only foods that are sweet, the use of sugar substitutes (with the doc-

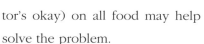

tor's okay) on all food may help solve the problem.

Difficulty with eating may also happen because of changes in physical abilities, making chewing or swallowing difficult. In such cases, reluctance to eat may be a spontaneous reaction, the only way the person can respond to the problem. Professional assistance is often needed in these situations, to determine which foods are safest to eat.

Only a careful examination by a knowledgeable doctor can determine a physical cause of eating difficulties. (There are even "swallowing clinics" that specialize in helping people overcome such difficulties.) If organic dysfunction is the source of the problem, caregivers need to rely on a combination of dietary changes and nutritional supplements to sustain the person.

Other possible solutions to reluctant eating include:

- Serve finger foods. A person with Alzheimer's may not know how to use or may have difficulty handling utensils.

- Limit the number of foods and utensils. It is sometimes helpful to serve one food at a time. If serving more than one, use divided plates to keep foods separated.

- Reduce distractions when eating. Turn off the television, limit the number of people in the room and keep conversation to a minimum.

- Allow the person with Alzheimer's to take as much time eating as he or she needs.

- Alternate solid foods with something to drink to keep the throat from becoming too dry.

- Provide ample drinking water to maintain hydration and prevent constipation. People with Alzheimer's may forget they are thirsty and become dehydrated. This can lead to medical and behavior problems.

- Make sure the person is in a comfortable chair and is fully upright, even if in bed.

- Remind the person to chew and then to swallow after each bite.

- Demonstrate chewing so the person can copy how you chew.

In the end stage of the disease, the person with Alzheimer's loses the ability to take sufficient food by mouth. This brings the caregivers face to face with decisions about prolonging life — should a feeding tube be used or is it better to keep feeding as well as possible by mouth? These types of difficult questions should be discussed before the crisis arises. It may even be possible, immediately after diagnosis, for the Alzheimer's patient to write out a living will that addresses such issues. But whenever the decision comes up, no one should expect to find the answer without the help and guidance of support groups, counselors, physicians and other professional caregivers.

Depression

Depression is common, especially in the early stages of Alzheimer's. It may be triggered by diagnosis of the disease, social isolation, awareness of the loss of physical or mental abilities, the loss of possessions or a home if there has been a change in surroundings, feeling unproductive and unsuccessful or changes in brain chemistry.

In the earliest stages of the disease, support groups, education about the disease and even individual therapy can help the sufferer come to terms with his or her condition.

It is also helpful for caregivers to emphasize that the person with early Alzheimer's still can exert control over his or her life by participating in decisions for the future. Each group of caregivers will have to make a determination of how much responsibility the person with Alzheimer's can assume.

For some people with depression, medication may provide dramatic relief. However, some researchers caution against using certain antidepressants that block production of the brain neurotransmitter acetylcholine, which is already reduced in dementia. Make sure the doctor is knowledgeable about the use of such medication for Alzheimer's patients.

ACTIVITIES

Activities are an essential tool in caring for a person with Alzheimer's. Anna Marie Landbo, Activities Coordinator, ManorCare Health Services, has developed a program of varied activities. "People with Alzheimer's respond positively to a structured routine and to a variety of scheduled activi- 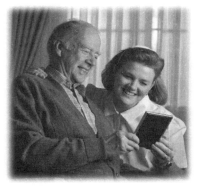 ties that keep the person active and stimulated," says Landbo. "Activities prevent boredom — a major cause of agitation. And just as important, activities instill a sense of accomplishment and boost self-esteem."

Activities are also important because they allow the person with Alzheimer's and the caregiver to spend quality time together doing something that is enjoyable.

Physical Activities

Keeping your loved one active helps expend pent-up energy and promotes good sleep patterns. "Some people will really go at it, and others will be more gentle," says Landbo. "But however they react, the physical activity is a release. You can bet they are having a difficult time with the disease — it gets them angry. Physical activity eases that and gives them the attention they need." Shared physical activities also allow you to have fun together — and that's important for the caregiver as well as the person with Alzheimer's.

Suggested physical activities:

- Ball toss. "I use a 16-inch punch ball because it floats and is easy to grab ahold of," says Landbo. Sitting or standing, you can throw the ball back and forth, increasing the distance between you as your loved one becomes more adept at throwing. Even if he or she isn't able to throw it to you, says Landbo, "punching it around can be very calming."

- Basketball. Use a soft, squishy ball. Place a laundry basket on the floor about three feet from the person. Take turns sinking a basket. Move the basket back as you play.

Thinking Activities

People with Alzheimer's like to solve problems and find solutions. It helps them recognize they have not lost all their former abilities. Thinking activities also help prompt memories, generate discussions, keep them oriented and give them a sense of accomplishment. Those people who previously worked with numbers often find pleasure in counting games or cards. Those who worked with words may enjoy flash cards or using the blackboard. Whatever thinking activities you do with your relative, it's important not to present him or her with mental tasks that are too demanding — that may produce agitation and anger. Simple "jobs" provide gratification and entertainment. Suggested activities:

- Matching cards, rolling dice, counting. These activities allow people with Alzheimer's to feel good about being able to do problem solving or basic math. "Large dice and cards with oversized numbers or pictures are helpful," says Landbo.

- Completing the phrase. You say things like, "a stitch in time..." and wait for the response. Questions can be easy or hard, depending on the severity of the dementia.

Household Chores

It's therapeutic for people with Alzheimer's to continue doing as much as possible for themselves. And they are more comfortable when they have a familiar routine to follow. So providing activities that allow them to continue former daily chores such as folding clothes, dusting or stacking papers can be very comforting and satisfying to them — it makes them feel productive and good about themselves.

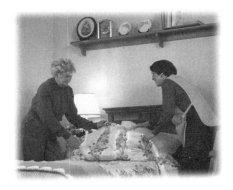

- Folding laundry. This is a particular favorite with many people with Alzheimer's since it is useful and reminds them of activities they used to do to take care of themselves. "You have to give credit and praise for whatever your loved one does," says Landbo. "If they want to sit all afternoon and fold towels, then let them do it."

- Basic chores such as dusting, setting the table, repairing a chair, watering the plants, making the bed or sweeping up. Although your relative may not do the task as proficiently as you would, you shouldn't criticize. If you have to repeat the chore yourself later, do so without comment.

Creative Projects

People with Alzheimer's are often drawn to crafts, painting and music. Such activities provide nonverbal people with a creative outlet for expressing emotions and ideas. They stimulate memories and help keep remaining skills sharp. These benefits all promote self-esteem. Suggested activities:

- Sing-a-longs. These are a wonderful shared activity. Familiar religious or holiday music, pop music standards and show tunes are all popular. "Get the sheet music so you have a copy of all the words or buy tapes that you can sing along with," advises Landbo.

You should start the song, allowing your loved one to join in as he or she wants. You may need to experiment for a while to find those songs that are most successful.

- Painting. You can choose chalk, pastels, watercolors, finger-paint, crayons, washable markers or colored pencils. Some people enjoy trying to draw what they see; others enjoy being left to do whatever they want. Don't force your loved one to accomplish a specific task — he or she should enjoy the process.
- Modeling clay or making collages. These activities are very popular with people who have Alzheimer's.

You may discover other activities that your loved one will enjoy. But whatever you do, advises Lisa Gwyther, MSW, "activities should be meaningful and pleasurable. The person should feel dignified and appreciated." Activities that work best are routine tasks and work-related projects that your loved one can associate with a dignified adult role. However, you may want to avoid projects that will remind your family member of how diminished his or her abilities are. "For example," says Gwyther, "Some artists don't enjoy painting because they can't meet their standards. But someone who never painted before may love it."

For additional information, the Alzheimer's Association offers a booklet on selecting activities at home.

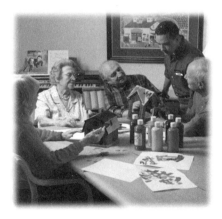

Emotional Stimulation

Through much of the disease, people with Alzheimer's still

feel the essential human emotions of love, longing for closeness, the need to give and receive affection, the pain of loneliness and isolation and the desire to share their feelings and be understood. At the same time, however, they may not be able to find the words or actions to express themselves. That can lead to depression, frustration and difficult behavior.

As a caregiver, you want to provide as many opportunities for emotional expression and sharing as possible — through touch, talk and shared activities. Some of the most effective techniques include:

- Arranging for the person with Alzheimer's to establish a regular relationship with a pet. Pets provide extraordinary benefits, allowing the person to express and receive unconditional love. Research has also shown that pets can relieve stress. If you do not have a pet, perhaps you can get one or work out an arrangement with a neighbor or friend to "borrow" their pet on a regular basis.

- Giving the person a gentle hand or foot massage. Touch is soothing and reassuring to everyone, but for some people with Alzheimer's it is especially comforting.

- Retracing old memories by looking through photo albums together.

- Singing or listening to music together. Many people with Alzheimer's find they remember old song lyrics quite well.

How to Handle...

DINING OUT

As Alzheimer's progresses, many families want to be able to take their loved one out to eat with the family. This can provide the person with welcome activity and help the family retain the feeling of a functioning unit, but it takes some thought and planning.

• Choose a quiet, well-lit setting. Go on off-hours.

• Inform the waiter that your loved one has special needs and assure him that you will take care of the person. But ask for his patience.

• Don't overwhelm your loved one with choices.

• Order easy-to-eat finger food. Avoid sauces or food that requires cutting.

• Bring a change of shirt or an apron from home.

• Don't worry about what other people think or how you look. You're there for your enjoyment, not to impress anyone else.

• If disruptive behavior occurs, don't argue or insist that you stay until you are finished. You may have to leave. Do so without rancor.

THE NEIGHBORS

Your neighbors may not be aware that your loved one has Alzheimer's or they may not know how to react. They can provide you with a helping network if you let them know what's going on.

One terrific solution is to write an open letter to your neighbors letting them know the situation, offering them reassurance and asking for their support. A sample letter may include: *(See next page)*

Dear Neighbors,

You may not know that my father, (name), who lives with us at (address) has Alzheimer's disease. As a result, he sometimes loses track of where he is. He may wander off and become lost or confused. You may see him in your yard, or walking by your house. He poses no danger to you, but may say things you can't make sense of or behave erratically. I would appreciate it if you could approach him gently and quietly. If you don't ask him too many questions but suggest that he come inside for a drink of water or let you bring him one, you may be able to detain him while you call me at (phone number). I will come and get him immediately.

This is a challenging disease, and it's not possible for me to police his activities all the time. I can't tell you how much I'd appreciate your help if the need arises.

Sincerely,

A Guiding Spirit

BY NILS LOFGREN

Nils Lofgren, musician and one of four sons,
has moved back to the East Coast
to be near his mother and his father, who has been
in a nursing home for almost two years.

"*M*y dad is one of the classic saints out of the movies. He raised us all with the be-kind-to-your-neighbors approach. My parents gave me so much.   I really owe my career to their support.   I know if they were against my being a musician I wouldn't have the success I've had. I'm lucky I get to spend this time with them.

"Dad was diagnosed with Alzheimer's when he was about 68, five years ago. He and my mother had recently retired. All the kids were grown and they were looking forward to some peace and quality time together.   The toll on both of them was enormous.   Mother struggled to take care of him but the disease wouldn't let him be still—he hardly slept.

After three years of basically no sleep, Mom realized her health was deteriorating from the stress. We had to move Dad to a nursing home before Mom's health decayed too badly.

"The whole family participated in making the decision to move him. But you could tell he was aware enough to realize that if it was going to help Mom, he wanted to do it.

"Lately, he's slipped quite a bit. He has trouble walking, talking, eating. But lots of times, I feel he knows exactly who you are and is happy to see you, even though he can't express it. Even on the worst days, he responds positively to the sense of safety he gets from being around family.

"His grandkids have all visited him—my three brothers have eight kids. They handle it well and that's a testimony to my brothers and parenting that comes from my Mom and Dad. His message was always, 'Be spiritual and don't be afraid of life,'—though I certainly get scared myself.

"Luckily, all of the brothers have been able to help. Tommy—he helps Mom out with her computer and keeping her files straight. Michael, who's a builder in the area, takes care of repairs around the house that Dad used to do. Even my brother, Mark, who lives in Minneapolis — he's got the expertise to handle a lot of the legal business that comes up. And my wife, Cis Rundle, whose work keeps her on the West

Coast, is tremendously supportive of my coming back East to be with my parents. So now I can see Dad three or four days a week when I'm in town. My brothers visit regularly, too.

"For any family facing this disease, I'd recommend that you gather all the information you can about Alzheimer's. It is very helpful to join support groups and meet other families who are struggling with it. If you hook into those a few times a month or more, it reduces some of the panic and fear. And I'd say you want to look very closely not only at the person with the disease but at the main caregiver to see what you can do to help them both. Since Dad moved into the nursing home, I think Mom's safer health-wise.

"Dad's always been very smart and very spiritual—a true saint on the planet. He lives his life like we're all supposed to. We've all gotten a lot from him. Even now I sense an emotional pain in my father. There's a part of him that's still being brave...trying to be the spiritual leader of the family and make the best of it.

"Mom has set a great example for all of us in learning how to handle Dad's illness. I'm very proud of Mom...and of Dad."

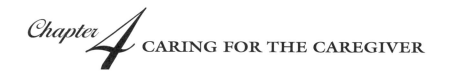

Chapter 4 CARING FOR THE CAREGIVER

*"There are always at least two patients when
dementia is the diagnosis.   From the moment someone
is diagnosed with Alzheimer's, the lives of those
closest to him or her will never be the same."*

~

Philip D. Sloane, MD, MPH

*W*hen a loved one develops Alzheimer's, your life changes. One day you're a wife or a husband or a daughter or a son. The next day you're a caregiver. That is not an easy transition, and particularly with Alzheimer's, the role can become overwhelming.

You may feel swamped by the day-to-day logistics of managing the disease. You may even feel inadequate or anxious when you can't figure out how to handle everything. The harder you try to cope, the more stressed you become. In the process of caregiving, you may forget to take care of yourself.

According to Lisa Gwyther, MSW, Director of the Family Support Program at the Duke Center for Aging, self-generated pressure to be the perfect caregiver often makes family members angry and frustrated. "It's important for you to give yourself credit for how you handle the situation. You do what seems best at the time and you can't expect more from yourself. If you expect to be the perfect caregiver, you're setting yourself up to become physically and emotionally exhausted. You'll end up taking it out on yourself and your loved one."

Alzheimer's is a long, slow disease. It is easy to lose sight of an important truth—taking care of yourself is an essential part of providing care for your relative.

CHALLENGES FACING THE CAREGIVER

Finding your emotional equilibrium when your loved one has Alzheimer's can be difficult. You're mad. You're sad. You're trying to figure out how to act. Watching your loved one slowly fade is heart-breaking. Coping with erratic behaviors may be frightening or embarrassing. Eventually the disease makes it impossible for the person with Alzheimer's even to recognize you.

If you're a member of the "sandwich generation," caught between taking care of children and parents, your responsibilities may be staggering. These days almost 60 percent of women with children work outside the home. If you're juggling the demands of a job, your children and caring for a relative with Alzheimer's, you want to be particularly aware of the dangers of caregiver burnout. You may become physically depleted, rundown, stressed out, without a moment in your busy day to recharge you own batteries. You may feel overused and unappreciated.

THIS IS TOUGH STUFF TO HANDLE

You don't need false encouragement. You don't want to be swamped with advice about how to provide care, and you sure don't want anyone telling you that if you just buck up, you can sail through the process without hitting rough spots. Yet all of us need support and advice at one time or another.

"Caring for someone with Alzheimer's is a roller coaster. Sometimes you feel strong, sometimes helpless and bewildered," says Gwyther. "That's only to be expected." Gwyther's approach is gentle and effective. "You don't have to figure everything out immediately," she says. "You don't have to make all the decisions about how to cope with providing care at once.

"In our research, the one thing that we recognized is most helpful to families is to stop assuming that it is a simple, straightforward process," says Gwyther. "In the best of all possible worlds, you wouldn't have to see your mother or father deteriorate, but you have limited choices, and nothing is going to make things the way they were."

Remember, above all, you're not alone, and, chances are, many other people in you situation feel the same way you do.

Why Being a Caregiver Is so Demanding

According to Dr. Philip Sloane, caring for someone with Alzheimer's is particularly difficult because:

* There are no medications available guaranteed to curb behavior problems or reverse the decline.

* In the early and middle stages, a person with Alzheimer's usually is physically healthy. He or she looks normal, but has problems with memory and thinking.

* People with Alzheimer's can remain ambulatory for many years. Coupled with their lack of judgment, constant supervision is necessary.

* Being a caregiver is a 24-hour-a-day job. The only way to get time off is to find someone who will relieve you.

* Caregivers are often too busy to remain connected to friends and community. This cuts them off from emotional support and helping hands.

HANDLING THE EMOTIONAL AND PHYSICAL DEMANDS

As a caregiver, you face two challenges – your own emotional upheaval, and the ever-changing physical demands of your loved one.

Emotionally you are faced with the process of grieving for your family member as he or she sheds his or her old life and personality. In so many ways the person with Alzheimer's may seem lost to you long before he dies. His or her personality and capabilities change. The person no longer fills the role in your life he or she used to.

Unlike the conventional process of grieving, caregivers don't move smoothly from one emotional stage to another, just as the person with Alzheimer's doesn't move smoothly from one stage of the disease to the next. Life becomes a series of jumps and starts — two steps forward, one step back. You can expect to experience sadness, depression, anger, resignation, even acceptance over and over again.

This can cause you to feel resentment, guilt and remorse. That's only natural. Pretending that it doesn't puts an enormous stress on you. And that's not good. You must be able to give expression to those feelings. The key is to find appropriate time, places and ways.

"It's easy to get lost in caregiving," says Dr. Sloane. Emotionally healthy people have many roles in their lives, but often caregivers begin to feel that caregiving is their only valuable role. In the long run, it is best to feel that you have some control over your life, or how at least some of your time is spent.

Physically, you will be challenged to find ways to manage behaviors, and to find the resources to fill your loved one's basic needs. In the later stages of the disease, you may lack the physical strength to help your relative with everyday tasks such as bathing, going to the bathroom or moving about with additional help. Specialists in Alzheimer's care all tell stories of caregivers who have driven themselves so hard that they land in the hospital or develop disabilities.

The stress on a caregiver is enormous and has serious repercussions. You can't be any good to your loved one if you are exhausted. You need respite and help.

SIGNS OF BURNOUT: A CHECKLIST FOR CAREGIVERS

1. Are you curtailing visits and phone calls with close friends? ❏ Yes ❏ No

2. Have you given up hobbies or activities that you have enjoyed for years? ❏ Yes ❏ No

3. Are you developing stress-related problems such as back pain, headaches, chronic feelings of fatigue and depression? ❏ Yes ❏ No

4. Are you coming down with colds, flu and other illnesses more than usual? ❏ Yes ❏ No

5. Do you have a short temper? Do you find you're getting mad in the checkout line at the grocery store? In traffic? With friends or family? ❏ Yes ❏ No

6. Do you have outbursts of anger at your loved one with Alzheimer's when he or she behaves erratically or becomes difficult? ❏ Yes ❏ No

7. Have you gained or lost weight unintentionally? ❏ Yes ❏ No

8. Do you have an unshakable feeling of despair or pessimism? ❏ Yes ❏ No

9. Are you crying "for no reason" or over minor problems? ❏ Yes ❏ No

10. Do you complain about lack of sleep or chronic insomnia? ❏ Yes ❏ No

If you answered yes to two of these questions, you are probably developing burnout. Yes to three or more questions indicates the need for immediate help from friends, family and social service organizations to ease your stress.

You are overtaxed, and your ability to provide quality care for yourself and for the person with Alzheimer's is in jeopardy. You may need to begin thinking about alternative care situations for your relative.

ASKING FOR HELP

There are few rules about providing care, but one that you should take to heart is: Ask for help.

The first place to turn is friends and family. Arranging for two or three short breaks a week will help you restore your energy. If you can expand that time, do so. But don't rule out possible assistance simply because it is only for short periods of time.

Participating in support groups made up of other caregivers is also tremendously helpful. You will learn how normal your feelings are and gather tips and tech-

niques for coping and caring.

Using social services, such as adult day care or at-home nursing services that are provided by the local, state or federal government at little or no cost, hiring an assistant or spending money on caregiving programs can help you cope with stress and fulfill the needs of your loved one. However, many caregivers are reluctant or unaware of how to use such resources. "Using social agencies or paid help can be difficult. Fear of spending money that might be needed later inhibits many people," says

Gwyther. "People are afraid that the future costs of the disease will be so great, that they don't want to spend money on services that will help them cope better today."

In addition, caregivers see respite services or day care, even when offered on a sliding scale so they aren't too expensive, as something they'd be doing for themselves instead of for their loved one. They don't want to spend money on themselves. But remember, a new friend or a new situation for your relative can be beneficial and fun.

Other obstacles to relying on social services or paid help include a mistrust of strangers, media stories of people being exploited or abused by home care workers and the feeling that, "No one can care for my Mom like I do." According to Gwyther,

most people turn to outside help only after they become disappointed in the availability or reliability of assistance from friends and family or when they are so overwhelmed they can't cope anymore.

As a caregiver, you want to recognize that easing your stress does help your loved one, because it keeps you strong physically and emotionally. It lets you avoid burnout.

You want to give yourself permission to ask for help before you reach such a crisis point. Relying on an ever-changing mix of family and friends, social services and support groups is the most effective. (For detailed information about support groups and social services, see the resource section at the end of the book.)

Bossing Around the Boss

BY SALLY AND JONI FORMAN

Two sisters talk about their struggle to overcome their family conflicts, which makes coping with their mother's Alzheimer's disease especially difficult.

Sally: "My sister Joni seems to have an easier time with Mom than I do. I don't have any luck persuading her to do anything. Mom was always in charge of her life. She and Dad had a very busy social schedule and she was the person whom all her friends depended on for advice and to organize activities. To this day, she's unwilling to give that up.

Joni: "When it came time for Sally and me to bring Mom to the nursing home, Sally and Mom got into a huge fight. Mom refused to get out of the car and started calling Sally every name in the book. Sally tried to explain to Mom what was going on — I remember she said, 'We tried to get you involved in the plans so you could make the decision, but you wouldn't cooperate.' I thought, 'Of course she won't cooperate, she is out of her mind.'"

Sally: "I thought I owed her the chance to be involved in the decision. It seemed like if we got her approval she would be happier."

Joni: "Sally told Mom she was going to tell the nursing home people that Mom refused to come in and that we were taking her home. But once Sally left, all I had to do was tell Mom I was going up to sit on a bench near the front door. When I did, she voluntarily came out of the car and joined me. It was just a few short steps to the inside. And she followed me gladly."

Sally: "Well, however we accomplished it, it was exhausting for everyone. We took her to her room that we had fixed all up. At first she didn't recognize that the furnishings were hers. But then she saw a picture of herself with my Dad and she wanted to know how that got in this strange room."

Joni: "After a few minutes the staff distracted her and we were able to leave quietly. I must say I was worried that Sally would say something to get her all agitated again."

Sally: "I know I don't have an easy time with Mom. That's why I wanted Joni there with me when it came time to move her in. I was scared after how she reacted when I took her around to visit different locations. She terrorized me. But since Joni lives out of town, I knew she could start off with a clean slate. I thought it was inspiration to pick Joni up at the airport, which Mom loved doing, and then drive straight to the nursing home. But you can't fool Mom. She really hated me that day. I thought she'd never get over it. But funny thing is now she doesn't really remember that anything happened."

Joni: "She's simply recreated her busy social life here with all the people in her living area. In fact, she's become the one everyone relies on if they need a shoulder to cry on. I love seeing her so involved and busy."

Sally: "I don't know. Sometimes I feel like she doesn't need me any more than she needed me when she was healthy. I mean I think this whole thing is a lot harder on me than on her. She just won't stop acting like she's the queen of the ball."

Joni: "How can she say Mom acts like the queen of the ball? I don't think we should be criticizing Mom, but Sally disagrees. We always get into disagreements about this. But never mind — we have got to stick together. Families can provide a lot of strength and comfort — maybe not exactly like we dream of, but good enough. Let's not make it so hard for the two of us. Hey, we're all we've got now. Let's prove that's plenty."

Chapter 5 FAMILY DYNAMICS

"My grandmother's Alzheimer's is more frustrating to
my mother and my sister than it is to me. They have a harder time
coping than I do, so I find myself overcompensating. I take on the
majority of interaction with Gram, because they get so upset."

⌒

Maggie K., 35, whose grandmother,

now 80, was diagnosed with Alzheimer's nine years ago

*W*hen one member of the family is diagnosed with Alzheimer's, it impacts every member—those who take on the role of primary care-givers, those who must handle new financial responsibilities, those whose hearts are aching with grief for their relative's emerging disabilities, even those who shy away from the tough responsibilities. Everyone is affected by the diagnosis, and in turn everyone affects the dynamics of the entire family group.

One person usually assumes the role of primary caregiver, while other family members accept varying responsibilities. As the primary caregiver, you may have to accept some slightly unpleasant realities about how your relatives do or don't lend a hand. . . but you're not stuck. There are well-established ways for creatively sharing the caregiving tasks that can ease your burden and help your relative with Alzheimer's receive the best care possible.

The basic plan allows you to work together as a family to provide quality care for your relative with Alzheimer's and to protect the primary care-giver from burnout. But there are no hard and fast rules about who should do what or how much time each person should devote. To devise a working plan, you have to let each person contribute to the best of his or her ability and to offer assistance that comes from individual strengths. Some people are better at handling the practical problems of finances or insurance. Others are best at offering a shoulder to cry on. Others may enjoy day-to-day caregiving. Each person is playing an important role and should be encouraged, not criticized, for doing what they can.

DEFINING THE ROLES

When the diagnosis is Alzheimer's, the entire family becomes involved in decisions about providing care. One member — a spouse, or a child who lives nearby — may automatically become the primary caregiver, even when other members would like to assume that role.

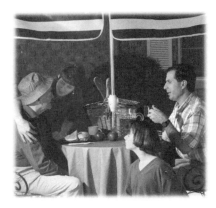

However it happened, if you have assumed the role of primary caregiver, it is now up to you to enlist the support of other relatives so that you are not overwhelmed by the role and so that, if they wish, they can participate in ways that express their love and concern. People who care would not want to be forced out of the picture. And there are plenty of "jobs" to go around.

Another relative may be adept at finance or legal matters and will take on those tasks. Several people may be delegated as respite providers, taking over for an hour or more during the week, or even taking the person into their homes for days or weeks at a time, so the primary caregiver can have a break.

"This is not a pie to be cut up evenly," says Merle Wexler, Director of Arden Courts Alzheimer's Assisted Living Facility in Potomac, Maryland. "That won't happen. Some people will take on more day-to-day responsibility. But that doesn't mean that there are not important contributions to be made by others.

TIP

Families will work together for the good of the person with Alzheimer's if they throw out the shoulds and look for the coulds. Don't get stuck on what you think someone should do. Instead, explore what he or she could do.

If your niece is away at college, for example, she can be the person who calls the primary caregiver every Saturday to check in. It's important to have someone to whom the caregiver can vent worries and complaints and explore new ways of managing difficult situations."

The division of family responsibility may cause problems and spark disagreements. Often family members have to deal with conflicting localities and obligations. The demands of family and work, geographic proximity and previous conflicts with the loved one can all make it hard to share the burden of care equitably. "But even when there are conflicts," says Wexler, "you want to reach out and find those people who are willing and able to assist you."

Too often a caregiver waits for others to offer to pitch in. Most people don't automatically volunteer; however, they may be eager to give what they can, but need for you to provide them with an opening. Remember, they, too, are bewildered by the disease and unsure of how to respond.

To enlist help from family, the first step is to have a pow-wow in person or by phone. Outline the areas of responsibility that need to be addressed:

- daily care;

- assistance — such as doing errands, making phone calls and respite for the primary caregiver;

- financial management of the current resources of the person with Alzheimer's and planning for the future;

- plotting out legal issues, such as power of attorney, custodianship and inheritance;

- coordination of and decisions about medical care;

- contact with local social services to see what assistance is available;

- discussion of future care situations for the person with Alzheimer's as the disease progresses and home care becomes difficult;

- exploration of insurance coverage and discussion of how to use it.

If it becomes difficult to enlist the help of family or there is confusion about how to handle the various tasks, a series of family meetings with Alzheimer's counselors, geriatric care managers, the patient's doctor, an attorney or financial planner and/or a social worker can provide clarity and ease tensions.

Once you have begun to unravel the problems of managing the life of someone with diminishing capabilities, you — as the primary caregiver — are still faced with enlisting enough practical day-to-day help that you don't reach burnout.

A SUPPORT NETWORK

To set up a support network for yourself, you need to reach out to those around you. The most important steps are:

- Ask for a helping hand.

- Talk to your relatives about their worries or fears about being responsible for a person with Alzheimer's. Answer their questions undefensively and suggest techniques for coping.

- Let them start off simply. Have them spend time with you and the person with Alzheimer's, adjusting to behaviors and seeing how you respond.

- Initially, don't leave a new helper alone with the person for too long. Even if all you do is take 20 minutes to run an errand or take a hot bath, you'll feel refreshed.

- Let your helper know how much it means to you to have a break.

- Explain that even if your loved one can't recognize the visitor or remember what they do together, people with Alzheimer's receive immediate benefits and pleasure. They thrive on affection, attention and respect. For example, if your neighbor takes your Dad to a ball game, it lifts his spirits and calms him, even if he can't follow the intricacies of the game or express his gratitude. A day later he may not remember that he went to the game, but that doesn't mean he didn't enjoy himself while he was there. Often people with Alzheimer's live in the moment — and there's no reason not to make that moment as pleasurable as possible.

One resident in a nursing home who's had memory loss for 10 years can still explain how important it is to her to keep contact with friends, even if her recollections are somewhat jumbled:

"I have friends that I made years ago. They still hold a precious place in my life. I frequently get letters from people I knew in high school. They say, 'We ran across so-and-so today and he says you're still alive and kicking and we wanted to get in touch.' That happens many times because I made many friends in my life. Sometimes they will stop over, after not seeing them for years. It's really a precious thing to renew a friendship."

How to Handle...

VISITS FROM FRIENDS OLD AND NEW

Worrying about how your loved one will behave around friends and relatives may cause you to stop inviting guests to visit. That severely compromises the quality of your life and increases the stress. Instead, you want to find ways to keep your network of contacts and to provide social interaction for the person with Alzheimer's as well.

You will have to decide what to do on an individual basis. Some friends and family members will be able to go with the flow better than others. Those who are easy-going don't need any special treatment. Ask them to come over whenever you feel like having them visit. Help them learn how to establish a new and appropriate relationship with your loved one. This may take several visits, but don't become impatient. After all, it's taken you some time to adjust to your new relationship and you're learning every day.

For friends and acquaintances who are not as likely to handle the unexpected gracefully, try the following:

• Have these people over during nap times or in the evening after your relative has gone to bed.

• Have friends and family over during activities you do with your loved one, such as gardening or cooking, and have them join in.

• Arrange for a helper or a home-care worker to watch your loved one while you have visitors.

• If your loved one becomes agitated when new people are introduced into the surroundings, don't expect him or her to visit with you. Let your loved one go into a separate room and watch TV, draw, fold laundry, etc.

THE GRANDCHILD'S VIEW

If your mom or dad has Alzheimer's and has moved in with your family, your children become part of the care process. No matter what their relationship has been with their grandparent, they may be confused, frightened or even angry about the new situation. Without meaning to, you may gloss over their developing problems, figuring that kids adjust. Unfortunately, this is not always the case, especially without some guidance and help from you.

"I remember the day my Pops ran outside and started screaming at nothing. Nobody could get him to stop," says Davey, 14, whose grandfather has lived with him for two years. "It was creepy.

"Now he's not always like that. I mean, I go up to his room and we watch TV. He likes old Westerns and that's cool. Some of my friends are used to him and they think it's sort of fun to talk to him. You never know what he will say.

"The funniest thing he ever did was one day in the grocery store, he started going up to everyone's carts and seeing all the junk they were buying and lecturing them. 'What are you wasting your money on this for? Don't you know this will rot your teeth?' I was laughing so hard. I mean he was right. But most people didn't see it that way.

"But I'll tell you. I hate it that he's sick. Mom says I shouldn't be selfish, but I had to give up my room and share with my brother. And you know, the fact that her father's sick, it makes her so sad. You start to think that getting old is, you know, kinda bad. How can a person be one way one day and then bam! Change like that? I've heard all the explanations. But it makes you think."

Children who live with a grandparent with Alzheimer's undergo their own crises. And their mothers and fathers, often overwhelmed with caring for the person with Alzheimer's, can miss the growing unhappiness or confusion that the children are feeling.

Some of the common problems that arise include:

- Lack of attention from one or both parents because they are on-call 24 hours a day, caring for the person with Alzheimer's.
- Parents skip special activities and events that are important to their children because they can't make arrangements for care.
- The person with Alzheimer's may direct his or her anger, frustration or paranoia at the child.
- Financial sacrifices or crowded living conditions may anger the child.
- Children may be too embarrassed by their grandparent's behavior to ask friends to come over to the house. They can withdraw socially and even become depressed.

How to handle this additional pressure:

- Include your child in family discussions about Alzheimer's disease and offer suggestions for responding to difficult behaviors. Even young children can understand that behavior problems are caused by an illness, not by their grandparent's intentionally willful actions.
- Allow your children to express their confusion, anger and worries. You'll be surprised what you can learn about their feelings if you listen.
- Make an effort to spend time alone with your child—even if it's only when you're running an errand or in the basement doing the laundry.
- Try to schedule regular family activities.
- Explain your parent's illness and behavior to your children's friends. It will make them less frightened and confused. Welcome visitors into the house. If you set a tone of acceptance and good humor about your parent's behavior, the kids will pick up on it.
- If your child is frightened of his grandparent with Alzheimer's, particularly if the grandparent directs his or her anger at the child, you must intervene to protect the child. Just saying, "Oh, ignore him," is asking a child to respond like a wise adult—and that's not fair.
- Instead, teach your child to respond calmly and gently as he or she walks away from the situation. And learn to rely on effective distractions — changing your parent's focus to an enjoyable activity. But intervening does take a gentle touch. As a caregiver, you want to keep the person with Alzheimer's agitation at a minimum.
- If your child is disrespectful because of having to give up a bedroom and/or getting less of your attention, the best way to get him or her to accept the tough reality is to tell the truth about what's going on and the choices that must be made. If you are loving toward your parent and your child, and explain that doing what's best for the family is ultimately more important than being able to go on a vacation or having one's own room, the child will come to accept the situation. If you, too, are resentful, then your child will probably follow your lead and remain angry about the circumstances.
- Locate or organize a children's support group in your area. For help, contact your local chapter of the Alzheimer's Association.

Learning to accept someone with Alzheimer's disease can be an enriching experience for young people and can help prepare them to deal with other challenges they must face in the future.

My Dad, the Strong, Silent Caregiver

BY *KEITH HERNANDEZ*

*Major league first-baseman Keith Hernandez
describes how caring for his mom took a dramatic
toll on his once-stoic father.*

"*T*he effect this disease has on the people around the
victim is devastating. In the last three years of my mother's life,
my father, John, aged dramatically. He went through a complete
transformation. Caring for Mom, who had been diagnosed with
Alzheimer's in 1980, was taking its toll. He was suddenly gray,
lined and wrinkled.

"Dad was very loyal. He had been married to my mom for 30
years. He was your typical John Wayne-type father who never
showed a lot of emotion. But I remember talking to him on the
phone, and he broke down crying. Dad and Mom had always
talked about traveling when he retired. Instead, Mom was in
diapers, and Dad had to change her.

"He didn't have much time left himself; he died, at 69, of cancer in 1991. But he did get help from the Alzheimer's Association. He did get strength and peace of mind from sharing his thoughts with other people who were struggling with Alzheimer's in their families."

Reprinted by permission of **People Magazine**.

Chapter 6
PROFESSIONAL HELP FOR HOME-BASED CAREGIVERS

"We battled with the local social service agencies for months,

but finally we got them to agree to reimburse us for occasional,

part-time, home health aide services.

Sometimes I wanted to give up. I figured I'd just do it all myself.

But now I'm glad I didn't. It makes me and my sister

much happier to have another person helping out."

⌐

Virginia C., 65, who has been caring

for her older sister for seven years

$\mathscr{N}$o matter how overwhelmed you feel by caring for your loved one with Alzheimer's, there is always hope and help available. Needing to turn to other people is no sign that you have failed or that you're shirking your obligations. Alzheimer's is a complex disease and makes huge demands on a caregiver. It's smart to enlist outside assistance.

WHERE TO TURN

You need a break – for a few hours, a weekend, a month. You need help to take care of your loved one's daily personal needs. You need to know you're not alone. There are many reasons why, as a home-based caregiver, you may turn to outside agencies and organizations, both public and private, for a helping hand. Below are the basic services that are available in most areas. You may want to take advantage of one or more of them at various times while you are the primary caregiver for your relative with Alzheimer's.

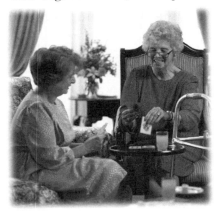

Adult Day Care

Adult day care programs are a cross between an activity center and a social club and offer supervision for the whole day or for a portion of the day. They can be a boon to both the caregiver and the person with Alzheimer's. Participating in a structured social situation often improves the quality of life for the person with Alzheimer's, while giving the caregiver a much-needed break.

Many senior citizen centers, churches, synagogues, hospitals, community centers and housing for the elderly run adult day care programs that accept people in the early or middle stages of Alzheimer's. Usually, transportation to a center can be arranged, and once there, your loved one will find friends and activities that can ease the isolation and frustration of living with the disease.

However, not all people with Alzheimer's do well in such environments. The daily shift from one location to another and the new stimuli and noise can overwhelm them, increasing agitation or behavior problems. But it's worth a try. The person usually adjusts to the new situation. And if it doesn't work this month, by next month your loved one may be better able to enjoy it.

In choosing an adult day care situation, you want to make sure that it meets certain standards:

- There should be a ratio of at least one supervisory person to every five to seven people with dementia. If the participants in the adult day care are a diverse group, special attention (and attendants) and activities should be provided for those with Alzheimer's.

- The area should be secure so that your loved one cannot wander off.

- The environment should be clean, cheerful and well-lit.

- Activities offered should include passive and active projects. Passive activities include watching movies, listening to records and looking at photos or slides. Active projects include bird-watching, field trips, arts and crafts, playing cards or board games and exercise routines. There should be a choice of activities. And there should be space and time for quiet periods.

- Meals should be nutritious, appealing to your loved one and presented in a way that makes them easy to eat.

- The overall noise level should be low.

- Personnel should be knowledgeable about and comfortable with people with Alzheimer's. Ideally, they should have some formal training in communication techniques, activities and behavior management as they apply to people with Alzheimer's.

Home Health Care Attendants

A home health care attendant may provide companionship, supervision and/or trained caretaking for a person with Alzheimer's. You may want to hire such a person to take care of your relative while you are working, to assist you while you are at home, or to come in for a few hours a week to give you a break. However, finding a home health care aide or companion who is caring, conscientious and dependable is not always easy. As the consumer, you must take responsibility for interviewing the person, checking references, establishing the rules of the house, making sure that rules are followed and dismissing the person if he or she does not prove to be satisfactory. That takes time and energy. You may want to have other family members help you with the hiring process. But once the worker is in your home, you must be sure that he or she is caring for your relative in a way that suits you.

To find the best qualified person:

- Go through established agencies or use references from friends and acquaintances who have firsthand knowledge of the person they are recommending. Sometimes, you can run an ad in neighborhood newsletters or newsletters from your house of worship.

- Check all references carefully.

- Arrange for the person to come for an hour or two (you should pay them for their time) so you can observe how they interact with your loved one.

- Never hire anyone sight unseen.

- Ask a family member or close friend to come over when you interview the person for the job.

- Be frank about the requirements of the job. Clearly explain the responsibilities you want the person to assume and the difficulties he or she may encounter in supervising your loved one.

- Whenever possible, look for someone with training in or experience with Alzheimer's.

Respite Services

Respite services are provided by caretaking facilities that accept people with Alzheimer's as temporary residents — for a few days, weeks or even months — so you can take a break from intense caregiving or attend to pressing personal or work responsibilities. Many caregivers find that using respite services so they can take a long-awaited vacation reenergizes them. They return happier with themselves, their jobs, their family and caregiving duties. Respite care also offers you a way to "try out" full-time placement in a long-term care facility.

Respite services are offered at many long-term care facilities, including nursing homes, and can be arranged on an individual basis by contacting the admissions director.

This service is not generally covered by federal and state reimbursement programs. If you need financial assistance to arrange respite care, some local chapters of the Alzheimer's Association have developed in-home respite programs or subsidiary funds. There are also many areas across the country that have developed their own

TIP

*W*here there is no question, there is no answer. Don't wait to have someone tell you what assistance is available. Ask everyone you talk to – every doctor or social worker you see, every association you call and every friend or acquaintance you talk with who has ever been a long-term caregiver.

respite services. The Family Caregiver Alliance in San Francisco is one example. To find out if there are such programs in your area, call everyone you can think of — from the local chapters of the Alzheimer's Association to visiting nurse services and state agencies.

Support Groups

Nothing is more essential or more helpful to the at-home caregiver than joining an Alzheimer's support group. Finding new friends who understand what you're going through and learning new ways of coping emotionally and physically with demands

of care offers great solace and eases stress. The Alzheimer's Association has local groups across the country. If there isn't a chapter in your area, contact the national or state headquarters for assistance in establishing one. Many nursing centers also offer support groups.

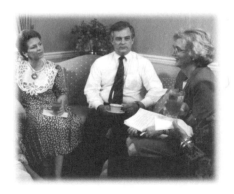

GETTING THE HELP YOU'RE ENTITLED TO

Once you decide to seek programs or people who can lend a hand with caregiving, you will want to explore the various public and private agencies that may cover all or part of the costs. Although such assistance is not always easy to obtain and may not provide all the help you need, it is available to those who are willing to track it down.

According to the Office of Technology Assessment's 1987 survey, physician's services, patient assessment, skilled nursing, physical therapy, home health aide services, homemaker services, chore services, paid companion/sitter services, home-delivered meals, telephone reassurance, transportation and adult day care are all available for people with dementia. (Changes in government programs may radically alter what's available, so for the latest information check with your state Medicare Office and Department of Aging.)

However, obtaining government reimbursement for these services can be difficult, and individual state agencies are often unpredictable and inconsistent in how they respond to such requests. In testimony before the Senate Subcommittee on Health, the director of a home health care agency stated: "A visiting nurse association in the Southwest was denied all visits to an 80-year-old Alzheimer's disease victim for March and April after being reimbursed for daily visits in previous months. Then the intermediary turned around after denying these two months and paid for two additional months of daily visits."

In contending with any bureaucracy, you should always remember that it's the squeaky wheel that gets the oil. Don't take "no" for a final answer. And carefully research all state regulations to be sure they are being applied fairly and according to the law.

Public Programs

Medicare provides acute medical care, medical supplies and equipment, part-time or intermittent skilled nursing care and part-time or intermittent home health aide services. Home health aide services include assistance with medications and exercise, personal care such as bathing and feeding, and homemaker services. To qualify for Medicare, however, the person must also need skilled nursing care — something that many people with Alzheimer's do not require.

Medicaid, a federal/state program, may offer slightly different services state to state, but can provide both acute and long-term care and may provide meals, transportation, adult day care programs and home health care services. However, the recipient must meet financial requirements. There is a Medicaid waiver program to allow states to increase flexibility in home health care services. Check to see if waivers are available in your state.

Supplemental Social Security Income provides monthly payments to the disabled that may cover home care and homemaker services. The amount of the stipend available and the willingness of services to accept the payments vary from state to state.

Services for the Aged under Title II of the Older Americans Act provides adult day care, home care, homemaker services and transportation. Contact your State Department of Aging for more information.

Private Assistance Sources

Many private organizations also provide support services or financial assistance for people with Alzheimer's who are living at home or with relatives. To find out what services are available in your area, contact:

- the local Alzheimer's Association;
- local Area Agencies on Aging;
- United Way;
- local hospitals to see what outpatient/caregiver programs they may have set up;
- local service groups such as the Lions Clubs or the Girl Scouts to see if they have, or are interested in starting an Alzheimer's care project;
- nursing centers.

PLAN AHEAD

Once you've recognized that you need a helping hand, it's a good time to start thinking about the day when your relative may move permanently into a long-term care facility. You don't want to have to scramble to find a facility when a crisis arises. Then, you'll be forced to take what's available, not what's best.

Many facilities have waiting lists, and there are financial plans and legal arrangements that you will want to make well in advance. Visit various facilities in your area or near other family members. Investigate their programs, staff training and cost. Get on their waiting lists, so you have options.

A Zest for Life

BY *JOELLEN*

*Joellen was a major in the WACS, a writer and mother
of two. She has been suffering from memory loss and
other symptoms for five years. After four years in a nursing
home, her enthusiasm for life has not been dimmed.
Despite the frustrations her disabilities pose, she can
still enjoy her environment.*

*W*hen did you first find out you had Alzheimer's?

***Joellen*:** "I first found out about my memory loss probably
about 10 years ago. It came up in a conversation with a doctor; I don't remember which doctor it was. He said I was suffering from dementia. A light loss of memory. I don't know
that any doctor has confirmed that and I still don't."

*When you were first diagnosed, did you make plans
for your future?*

***Joellen*:** "I don't remember it being that cut and dried."

***What about your husband? Did he help you
make plans?***

Joellen: "We made out wills and all that kind of thing. It
was kind of alluded to when we were making our wills and
things like that. You know, if it continues that you lose
memory, so on. I really didn't believe it, especially when you
are as decisive a person as I was. I was always on top of
everything. I had responsibility for people beginning in 1924
with a job with the WPA and then later on... what did I do?
I had the WPA job, I don't remember what else. I had
responsibility because I was always the leader. I was a
WAC major."

What changes in your abilities have you noticed?

Joellen: "It's a very gradual thing. It wasn't until my
husband and I were doing our wills... I agreed and understood that his was sort of a factual kind of remembrance
and mine was..."

Have you been aware of changes lately?

Joellen: "That's a strange question, because how do you
know? You can't remember. Friends, I remember some of
them with jagged memories. That's just about as fair a
description as anything I know."

Has your behavior changed?

Joellen: "I don't feel I behave differently. I'm still as belligerent and decisive and definite as always."

What does it feel like when you forget information?

Joellen: "It makes me furious. 'Cause I don't believe it. I think I can drag them to the front."

What advice would you offer to another person with dementia?

Joellen: "Write everything down."

What would you tell family members?

Joellen: "Don't expect too much."

When you look at your life, what things give you pleasure?

Joellen: "Living. Living is a pleasure."

Chapter 7

ASSISTED LIVING, NURSING HOME AND SPECIAL CARE UNITS: WHY, WHEN AND WHERE

"After five years of caring for Dad, my mother was worn out.
Her health was failing. She couldn't handle my father's
physical needs. But convincing her that they
would both be better off if he went into a nursing home
was the hardest thing my sister and I ever had to do."

Sally R.

*T*here are no rules to follow that will tell you when it's the right time to place your loved one in an assisted living, nursing home or special care facility. Every caregiver must make the decision based on the unique realities of the situation.

For some families, the best decision is to keep the loved one at home as long as possible, relying on at-home nursing and assistance or enlisting friends and family to share the tasks. For others, it becomes clear early on that the person with Alzheimer's and the caretaker will have a better quality of life if the care is provided in a nursing home or supervised situation.

The physical strength of the primary caretaker, the demands of work and family, the needs and behaviors of the person with Alzheimer's, financial resources and the ability of the caregiver to provide security and stimulation to the person with Alzheimer's are all factors that must be weighed. "In general, I think there is no one right place for a person with Alzheimer's disease," says Duke's Lisa Gwyther, MSW. "But placement in a residential care setting is not an indication of failure."

As heart-wrenching a decision as it can be, a care facility is often the most appropriate option.

MAKING THE DECISION

Alzheimer's disease often involves parting, slowly and painfully, from your loved one. Most caretakers long to hold on to their relationship with the person with Alzheimer's as long as possible. Having him or her at home helps retain some sense of the way things used to be. That's why if it comes time to move your loved one into another care situation, the wrench can be terrifically upsetting. Hopefully, you will find the wisdom and strength to make the decision when it is best for both your loved one and for you.

It may be difficult to admit that despite your best efforts and love, you simply cannot provide the quality care you want to. You may find that there are many emotional obstacles to making such a choice:

- Love and loyalty may make you determined to provide care yourself. In fact, some spouses have made a vow not to place the other in a nursing home.

- Guilt may make you ashamed of your desire to shift the hardship of providing care to others.

- Worry may make you afraid that your loved one will not be happy or well taken care of by "strangers."

These are difficult feelings to overcome. You can't simply wish them away. But there are some questions to consider that might help you make an objective evaluation of your situation and ease your mind about "doing the right thing."

TIP

Deciding to place your loved one in a long-term care facility shouldn't be the last resort – it can be the best resort. Such a move can improve your relative's care and safety...and provide an environment where he or she can thrive.

Can you provide an unrestricted and stimulating environment?

During the early and middle stages of the disease, if you find it necessary to restrict your loved one's freedom of movement in order to prevent accidents or wandering, it may be best to move him or her into a supervised living situation. This may be your only choice if you have to leave the house to work, and family and friends are not available to provide supervision or you don't have the financial resources to provide day care or hire home care helpers. But, trying to protect your loved one by locking him or her in a room or confining him or her to a bed or chair causes a whole new set of problems. For all your love and hard work, your loved one is suffering. Restriction is humiliating, frustrating and frightening. Lack of stimulation is depressing and boring. That can make a person with Alzheimer's angry and agitated, and new behavior problems can develop.

In such a difficult situation, it may become clear that moving your loved one to a care facility will benefit both of you.

Is your loved one comfortable remaining in his or her old environment?

Some people are overwhelmed by being in their own environments and not being able to manage what they used to do. They feel like failures and obsess about not keeping track of things. They're afraid that in some way they are not living up to expectations. Sometimes they do better in a less demanding environment with fewer reminders of their previous way of living.

Are your loved one's behavior problems wearing you out and making you angry?

Burnout is a serious problem for caregivers. It compromises your health and the quality of care you can provide. You may think you should be able to rise to every challenge, always finding the right solution to each new crisis. No one can. Sometimes it simply becomes too much. Everyone has his or her own threshold. We each do what we can, and that is all we can ask of ourselves.

The physical demands of providing care may also exceed your abilities — your husband may simply weigh too much for you to help him bathe or go to the bathroom. Agitated behavior may imperil you. Your loved one may hit or shove you.

Sometimes, if you are pushed to your limits by physical or emotional demands, you find yourself lashing out. You may find that you are becoming angry or irritated over the slightest problem, yelling at your loved one, criticizing him or her, losing your temper.

Then it's time to step back and take a long look at the benefits of moving your loved one into a care facility. Once you have been able to repair your frayed nerves, you will be able to reestablish a much more loving relationship. You'll find renewed inner strength, so you can participate in the care of your loved one in his or her new home.

Are you having health problems?

Many caregivers are age 50 or older or have health problems, and the stress and physical demands of caring for someone with Alzheimer's leads to serious health problems. Too often the caregiver dies before his or her spouse with Alzheimer's does. You don't want to drive yourself so hard that you can't help your loved one. Not only may the hardships of caregiving compromise your health, but if you become ill and your loved one cannot help you, that imperils you both.

"We have a woman here now who was terribly traumatized when her husband had a fatal heart attack in front of her and she couldn't do a thing to help," says Anna Marie Landbo, ManorCare Health Services. "That made her extremely disoriented and depressed. When she came here she jabbered into a mirror she carried everywhere with her. She was very withdrawn. It was difficult to get her out for meals. She clung to a teddy bear. But I

worked with her for a long time, and little by little she calmed down. She set the mirror aside, and she would leave her teddy bear in her room and come out for meals. She began participating in group activities. She'd speak in two- or three-word sentences. It was wonderful to see her blossom. Her niece, who was her caregiver after her husband died, has said many times that it was the right thing to place her in our facility."

Remember your goal for your loved one — to provide as high quality a life as possible for him or her at each stage of the disease. If the way for you to achieve that goal is to transfer daily caretaking duties to a facility that specializes in the care of people with Alzheimer's disease, then that's the best choice.

STAYING INVOLVED

Moving your loved one to a care facility does not have to — in fact, should not — mean that you will no longer be a vital part of the caring process. Your participation in a care facility is vital for your loved one's well-being. The professionals who will attend to the daily routine of care need your help.

In addition, staying involved will provide you with an ongoing connection to your loved one. You may even find that freed from the daily stress and physical duties of caregiving, you'll be able to relax more so you can provide more emotional support and enjoy the time you spend together. Your role may shift — but it can become even stronger and more beneficial than it was at home. "You may feel guilty and think you're abandoning your loved one," says Landbo, "but I have found that after a short while family members tell me, 'I made the right decision.'"

(For more detailed information on how to work with the new caretaking staff, see Chapter Nine: Partnership for Care.)

FINDING A QUALITY CARE ENVIRONMENT

If you decide that it's time to make the move, you're faced with finding a situation that provides the environment you want for your loved one.

The type of facility you choose is not as important as the quality of care provided. And quality care results from a knowledgeable, concerned staff committed to providing individualized attention and to allowing families to stay involved in the care.

The facility's philosophy and goals should encourage resident independence and functioning and ensure dig-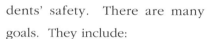nity and individual expression. There should be minimal use of restraints and medication, while ensuring residents' safety. There are many goals. They include:

- reducing confusion and agitation;

- maximizing independence;

- monitoring physical abilities;

- creating a pleasant experience.

"The facility doesn't have to be a specialized unit to provide good care," says Philip D. Sloane, MD, MPH. "However, it should have staff who are trained in Alzheimer's care. It should offer specialized programs tailored to the needs of people with Alzheimer's, such as an in-house day program of activities and supervision suited to the disease stages of each resident. You want a staff who gets to know your loved one's individual strengths and needs," says Dr. Sloane.

Talk to the director. See if he or she seems to understand the disease and says things that make sense from your experience. Dr. Sloane also suggests that families looking at a facility should ask many questions, including the following ones.

Is the staff well qualified?

Assess the staff. Look for the presence of a full-time Alzheimer's director and/or program coordinator. All staff members should receive ongoing training in caring for people with dementia. Lastly, there should be a high staff-to-patient ratio around the clock, and a consulting medical specialist should make regular visits.

Are staff members enthusiastic about their jobs?

Talk to staff members, including aides and meal service personnel. See if they are enthusiastic about their jobs and concerned about the residents. Find out if there is consistent staffing so residents can build relationships with the aides and nurses.

Are there individualized care plans?

Ask about how the staff structures each resident's care. There should be individualized care plans created with the input of family and an interdisciplinary care team. The plan should change as resident needs evolve.

How is the design of the facility?

Take a critical look at the environmental design of the facility. The facility should be safe and

TIP

"The strongest first impressions of a facility often involve its appearance and leadership. But the staff providing day-to-day care will be the most important in the long run," says Dr. Sloane.

secure. It should be clean and orderly. The floor plan should make it easy to get around. There should be bathrooms adjacent to most activity areas. There should be regular access to a safe outdoors environment. There should be several public rooms, so that more than one activity can go on at once.

Are meals nutritious and tailored to individual abilities?

Have a meal with the residents. Taste the food and gauge how the residents are treated as a group. Investigate how meals are planned — they should be tailored to the nutritional needs and abilities of each resident. Specialized utensils should be available to make it easier for residents to feed themselves. In addition, between-meal snacks should be served several times a day or (better yet) available at all times.

Are residents happy?

Spend time observing residents. Are they well-groomed? Are they occupied and supervised?

Are there activities? Inquire about activity programs.

A good facility provides paid activity therapists daily, including evenings and weekends. The activities should include active and passive programs, be of short duration and take place in large groups, small groups and one-on-one. Activities should be success-oriented, focusing on what residents can still do, rather than what they can't.

In many facilities, says Dr. Sloane, "residents cluster around the nurses' station. This is always a sign that there are not enough structured activities being offered."

THE CHOICES

There are four residential options available to people with Alzheimer's disease — *supervised living, assisted living, skilled nursing* and *Special Care Units.* Choosing the appropriate option/setting will depend on their specific needs. How much help do they need with activities of daily living, such as dressing, bathing, eating? How much supervision do they require? Are they somewhat independent? Do they need skilled nursing care? Each residential option is designed to offer as much independence as the resident can responsibly manage.

Supervised living allows a house- or apartment-like environment with supervision to provide safety and security. Caretakers check in on residents, provide assistance arranging for household maintenance tasks, make arrangements for transportation and help with other tasks as they arise. Many retirement communities these days offer residents the chance to move from their original homes into such supervised living areas.

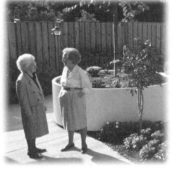

Assisted living facilities provide increased supervision for frail elderly who want to remain in a homelike environment and don't require full-time nursing care, but who require help with daily tasks. Many such facilities provide group social activities, communal eating areas, organized activities and excursions, housekeeping assistance and help with personal tasks such as dressing, hair styling or bathing.

Springhouse® facilities of Manor Care Health Services, for instance, offer assisted homelike accommodations combined with daily personal care assistance, meals and social activities for those unable to live independently, but who do not require full-time nursing care.

These days, realizing that people in the early-to-middle stages of Alzheimer's disease could benefit from living in a more residential environment, assisted living facilities are being designed specifically for people with dementia. For example, ManorCare Health Services' Arden Courts® provides residential living for people in early-to-middle stages of Alzheimer's. In surroundings designed to accommodate personal furnishings and possessions, the person with Alzheimer's is able to enjoy the feeling of living on his or her own while being able to participate in activities tailored to his or her skills and interests, such as sports, music appreciation, card games, art, cooking and gardening. Residents are also encouraged to continue performing daily tasks, such as light housekeeping, setting the table, watching television and getting the mail.

Skilled nursing facilities (nursing homes) provide a third option — they offer round-the-clock supervision and care from licensed registered nurses and other staff members. Nursing homes are appropriate for people whose condition has begun to affect their physical well-being or who have developed other medical problems in addition to Alzheimer's.

The quality of care in nursing homes across the country varies widely. However, there are many general nursing home situations that provide quality care and a supportive environment that benefits patients and encourages the continued participation of caregivers. Many Manor Care Health Services nursing facilities, offer a Laurel Day® care program, a special in-house day program for residents who have Alzheimer's. This enables them to receive the skilled nursing care they require while also providing them with specially designed activities that keep them active and stimulated.

Louise, 72, has been living in a nursing center for three years. Although she misses her former life, she is definite about how much she enjoys her new surroundings and the companionship of new friends. "My living arrangements are very nice. You meet new people, which inspires your morale. I have enjoyed being here and learning what I have learned. I have a very congenial roommate. We sort of help each other. If we are upset, talking helps. I've been happy here, because I have people who are good friends around me and we talk and discuss things that are bothering each one of us. It helps a lot to talk. We support each other."

Finally, many nursing centers have designated and secured wings called **Special Care Units** (SCUs). They are designed exclusively for people with Alzheimer's who require increased nursing care and general supervision to maintain their quality of life. These units offer the highest level of care. As you evaluate facilities, you might use the standards of ManorCare Health Services' Arcadia® unit as yardstick to measure the quality of other locations.

In an Arcadia unit, residents are surrounded by a supportive and well-trained staff of specialists who provide activity and therapy programs that keep residents at their highest level of functioning. The environment is designed for safety so that there is no restriction on movement or social interaction. A sense of independence and dignity is preserved. A staff made up of nurses, aides, housekeepers, dietary technicians and activity coordinators works together to tailor the daily routine to the needs of each person. The staff is supported by consulting medical doctors, physical therapists, occupational therapists and behavioral

scientists. Special architectural designs, such as fully enclosed courtyards, allow for safe and uninhibited enjoyment of the outdoors, and calming colors, carpeting and soft, nonglare lighting work to minimize distractions and agitation. Visual cues such as pictures on bathroom doors and walls, photographs on bedroom doors and contrasting colors on walls and doorways also help to keep residents oriented.

And family involvement is paramount. From the beginning, family members should be involved in care planning, social activities and developing responses to their loved one's ever-changing needs.

Jane, who has been living in a nursing center for three years, sums up the benefits of living in such a facility. "It's very much like a sorority or dormitory, but we have more fun."

BENEFITS OF PLACEMENT IN A RESIDENTIAL/NURSING FACILITY

Staff who care for dementia patients often report that new residents show marked improvement in behavior and well-being. The most common improvements are:

- a decrease in wandering;
- less frequent agitation;
- a decrease or absence of screaming episodes;
- a decrease or absence of medication;
- better orientation to surroundings;
- improved eating habits or weight gain;
- a decrease in socially unacceptable behaviors;
- less depression;
- better sleep patterns;
- an increased sense of humor;
- a more happy, relaxed appearance;
- formation of friendships;
- reduction or elimination of incontinence.

CRITICISM FROM FRIENDS AND FAMILY

Occasionally, other family members or friends are critical of a decision to move your loved one into a care facility. This can be frustrating, insulting, and guilt-provoking. You don't need them to make your life any more complicated than it already is.

Your first impulse may be to tell them to mind their own business. But this may alienate those very people who at other times have provided you with support and understanding. Besides, if they love the person with Alzheimer's too, it is their business. They deserve to understand why a care facility is the best choice.

To help you handle their criticism, take a deep breath and ask yourself what's making them so critical:

- *Have you "protected" them from the more difficult aspects of caring for your loved one?*
  If so, they simply may not understand what has been involved. Perhaps it is time to share your feelings with them. Let them in on how being a caregiver has affected you. They care about you and don't want to see you become burned-out or ill.

- *Are they feeling guilty over their own inability to step in and take over care?*
  Offer them reassurance that your loved one would not be best served by moving in with another family member. Take the time to explain the difficulty you — or anyone else — would have meeting your loved one's current needs for supervision, behavior management, medical care and/or physical assistance.

- *Are they out of date in their thinking about the kind of care a nursing home can provide?*
  In the past, nursing homes were not as well regulated as they are now, and medical science was not as knowledgeable about how to best provide for people with Alzheimer's. Assure them that things have changed and suggest that they come with you to see the facility so that they won't be unnecessarily worried about what will happen to your loved one.

If you have done your best to ease your friends' or families' concerns and they still disagree with your decision, remember, as primary caregiver you know best what your loved one needs. You have provided quality care for months or years, and moving the person with Alzheimer's to a nursing home is a continuation of that loving attention.

The Best I Could

BY *SHELLEY FABARES*

*Her mother's increasing frustration over not being able
to communicate and her own struggle to let her mom know
how much she cherished her continue to haunt actress
Shelley Fabares.*

"*M*ost people are close to their mothers, but my Mom
and I had a truly special bond. She had to act as my
guardian on the set of The Donna Reed Show when I was
working and my Dad, James, was away a lot during the
week, so I spent tremendous amounts of time with her.

"The first clear sign of the disease came in 1984. That was
the year I married Mike Farrell, and Mom, who was 73 at the
time, refused to buy us a wedding gift. Her reason makes no
sense. It was so strange. She did other strange things, too.
Smokey, my older sister, and I invited Mom to go to a movie.

She said, 'No, I won't go to that movie. That movie stars a short person. And I hate short people.' I thought, 'What? Who are you? I don't like you!' The company that Mom worked for noticed the change, too. They kept lessening her responsibilities, thinking maybe they had been pushing her too hard.

"Smokey and I decided to take Mom to the doctor. We wound up seeing neurologists, psychologists, specialists of many kinds. We felt it was our duty to find out what was wrong. None of the doctors, though, could tell us.

"Finally in 1989, the doctors told us that Mom had multi-infarct dementia (deterioration of mental abilities caused by multiple strokes) and probable Alzheimer's.

"Mom had to leave her job, and we hired a 24-hour-a-day live-in caretaker. One day in 1990, I got a frantic call from Mom's caregiver. The woman had been out of the room for just a moment and returned to find Mom gone. We found her in the middle of a busy street, yelling and flailing her arms at the people who were trying to help her. At that point we had to place her in a nursing home.

"Often in the last years of her life, I told her how much I admired her. I told her that I regretted it had taken so long for me to look at her as a friend and not just my Mom. But by then it was really a monologue, not a dialogue. Mom was 81 when she died in September of 1992. I tell myself I did the best that I could."

Reprinted by permission of *People Magazine*.

Chapter 8 MAKING A SMOOTH MOVE

"When it comes time to make the move, you want to try to
set your loved one up in a homelike environment
that helps him or her feel secure and comfortable.
Familiar objects can be helpful,
but the atmosphere and sense of familiar comfort
are more important than the specific possessions
they may bring to the facility."

⤸

Philip D. Sloane, MD, MPH

*P*lanning for and going through moving day presents a new set of emotional challenges and practical considerations. You can handle them if you are well-organized and give yourself ample time to prepare.

That doesn't mean that the move will be easy for you. Even though it is a positive step, you may be sad that you have had to come to this conclusion. But you should focus on the fact that as you face this new phase in your life, you and your loved one will continue to share an unshakable bond, and your role as a caregiver remains essential. Remember, you are not saying good-bye.

HOW TO TELL YOUR LOVED ONE

Deciding how and when — or even if — to tell your loved one that there's a move coming up depends on your assessment of his or her ability to deal with the information.

In the earlier stages of the disease, you will probably want to discuss it, giving your loved one the respect and dignity that comes with participating in this important life decision. You may even want to involve the person in choosing the home.

Telling a relative with Alzheimer's about a planned move does not always go smoothly. You may encounter resistance and resentment. As heartbreaking as it is to hear your loved one's protests, they should not make you change your mind.

"You want to do what is good for your loved one," says Dr. Sloane, "and that is not necessarily what he says he wants."

You may want to concentrate on the fact that even if your

relative is unhappy about the move, once he or she is in an environment that offers security, freedom of movement, social interaction and interesting activities, he or she will settle in comfortably. And you should reassure the person with Alzheimer's that the move does not mean that you don't love her or that she will never see you.

Timing is important, however. At certain times, your loved one may be more agi-

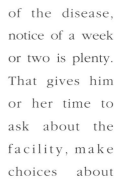

tated, paranoid or angry. Changes in environment, the presence of new faces and loss of familiar surroundings can all increase anxiety. It may not be possible to eliminate the negative reactions to change entirely, but you do want to diminish them as much as possible. That's why it's

smarter, if possible, to make the move when the person is in a relatively calm period.

When you do tell your relative that he or she will be moving to a care facility, offer an explanation in a straightforward way. And don't bring up the subject too far in advance. In the early stages of the disease, notice of a week or two is plenty. That gives him or her time to ask about the facility, make choices about what he or she wants to take, even visit the facility if that is appropriate. You can schedule an appointment with a social worker or the doctor to get help with answers to questions and worries.

You may want to say something like: "Mother, next week we're going to take a drive to a place where you are going to live. It's got lots of other people your age for you to spend time with and you'll be able to do a lot of activities that you don't get to do now. I'll be going with you that day, and afterwards I'll see you there all the time."

Listen to what your family member has to say. Don't overload him or her with information. If he or she mentions not wanting to leave behind certain possessions, offer reassurance that the treasures will be moved too. If that is not possible, assure the person with Alzheimer's that there will be many things to enjoy in the new place.

In later stages of the disease, however, you may determine that it is neither necessary nor wise to tell your relative that the move is going to happen. Instead, you may simply want to wait until moving day to mention it — he or she may not even understand or react.

A CALMER PLACE

"My husband doesn't understand that he's moved," says Patricia, who placed her husband of 40 years in a nursing home. "He's just as happy there, or maybe even happier, because the grandkids aren't running in and out. There's no commotion. He's more settled and has adapted very well. He doesn't ask to come home."

In the middle of all this, you should not overlook another important person who deserves sympathy and understanding — you.

You may be sad, angry or depressed about giving up your role as primary caregiver. For husbands and wives who, after decades of marriage, will now be living alone, this can be a particularly difficult transition. It is vital that you find a way to remain in as close contact as possible. Set up visiting schedules, arrange transportation, participate in the care-planning and activities in the facility.

MOVE-IN DAY

Packing up possessions and moving furniture should be done as close to the move as possible. Consider packing personal effects and treasures immediately before you leave so that your loved one doesn't become agitated or confused by the changes. If you must disrupt the home environment ahead of time, anticipate that you may have to cope with challenging behaviors. Try to have friends, family or home-care helpers on call for several days to lend a hand. To minimize agitation, if you must pack in front of the person with Alzheimer's disease you may want to have a friend or relative keep him or her distracted while you complete the task.

When deciding what possessions to move:

- Choose photographs from the past and current ones of friends and family.

- Select a favorite, comfortable chair, if room permits.

- You may want to take a pillow and blanket from home, so the sleeping environment is familiar.

- Bring games or crafts that he or she enjoys.

- Pack favorite clothing, slippers, nightgowns and pajamas.

- Select special mementos and objects to decorate the room.

You may be questioned over and over about what is happening. Try to remain patient and answer the question directly. "We are moving you to a new house where you'll meet new friends. I'm coming with you." If you can remain calm and collected, it will go a long way to making the whole process easier for everyone.

Setting Up the Room

If you are moving furniture from home or having new furniture delivered to the location, have it all in place when you arrive at the facility. You can then help your loved one arrange pictures and place mementos on the dresser and tables so that there is a feeling of continuity with home life. However, re-creating the home environment is not essential.

Persons with Alzheimer's disease often don't remain as attached to a specific personal item as families anticipate. More important is to replicate the feeling of privacy and familiarity.

Patterns are important to make a move go smoothly. Ideally the bed should be oriented in the same way toward the window or bathroom as it was at home. This is not crucial in the long run, however, because the new environment will gradually become familiar.

It is also important for families to realize that in an Alzheimer's facility most possessions are communal. No matter how conscientious the staff is, roommates and other residents will "borrow" each other's possessions, clothes and trinkets. Although they are usually easy to retrieve, items of real value should be marked with the owner's name or left at home.

Saying So Long

When it comes time to leave your relative's side, work with the nurses, aides and activity director to make it as smooth as possible.

They should help involve your loved one in an activity — a game of ball toss, a meal, a walk down the hall, a conversation with one of the staff members. Distracting attention from the farewell will help both of you cope more easily.

If Only I Could Tell You

BY FIVE RESIDENTS OF AN ASSISTED LIVING FACILITY

*Five friends share their thoughts on the benefits of living in
an Alzheimer's assisted living facility and demonstrate how
their lives have improved.*

*These women, ages 65 to 78, come from diverse
backgrounds — one was a bookkeeper, one was an editor,
two were teachers, another a telephone operator — yet they
have found companionship, affection and fun in
their growing friendships.*

Belle, a teacher, who, as her daughter says, always ran
the show and had lots of friends, was furious about making
the move a short six weeks before. Now she says: "I've met
so many new people. They are very interesting and we
spend a lot of time doing things together. Some of the girls
are having a harder time, but I help them. I particularly like
the discussions we have about the news. And we're always
arguing about the movies we see. I like it here."

Rene, a former telephone operator who had not spoken a
word for more than six months before coming to the facility,
has, after three weeks, become the most talkative of the group.

She's got a sly humor and loves to make side comments about what she observes.

"This is an unusual place. I got my hair done today and my nails. The woman who does it is very talented. My room is okay; I don't have to work so hard to keep it clean. But I do get to do a lot of things like painting pictures. You get to relax. It used to be so confusing. Now we get along better."

Julia, an accomplished teacher and music lover, wonders about Alzheimer's and what it means for her. "Did they talk about this disease when we were younger? It seems to me they did. But still no one can tell me much about it. But here I will be able to find out. And I hope I won't have to worry about it so much. With all these friends around, you know, you can keep up on things."

Marcia, an elegant woman whose tales of her teen years make everyone laugh, finds acceptance. The most confused of the group, the other women encourage her to talk about her former life as an editor and show no impatience when she repeats the same story over and over. She no longer worries about whether she's being socially correct, and has expressed much less frustration and agitation since she arrived two months ago.

"There are wonderful people here. Did I mention my neighbor when I was young? Do you know him?" she asks the group. "We do now," someone answers, and everyone laughs. "You're laughing at me because you know him from my telling you so often," she says. "Well I'm going to tell you again." And everyone claps their hands and says, "Okay."

Gretchen was a bookkeeper in her family business for 40 years and misses the work. Everyone in the group seems to realize that she's having a hard time accepting that she can't have a job anymore. Belle is particularly gentle with her, letting her cry on her shoulder and offering suggestions. Others ask her opinion about TV news stories that involve economics. No matter how badly she's feeling, she perks up right away. "I guess you could clean up the deficit," says Rene. "You bet. Right away," answers Gretchen.

Chapter 9
PARTNERSHIP FOR CARE

*"I was so afraid that Mother wouldn't miss me when
other people were taking care of her.
But since she's been in the special unit, I've found that
I have a lot to do with her care. And even if she doesn't
know who I am sometimes,
we can enjoy each other's company."*

᠆᠆

*Esther F., whose 78-year-old mother
moved into a special care facility after living with her for six years*

When your loved one moves into a care facility, your importance as a caregiver does not end, it evolves. Once the burden of day-to-day care is lifted, you can concentrate on providing emotional support. And you become a partner with the professional care team to help create the best care for your family member.

Families may establish their own level of involvement, but often they can do more than they realize. Their role remains extremely important.

―――――――――

WORKING WITH THE STAFF

Every nursing home facility is required to set up a care plan for each resident. This covers medical attention, activities, a nutritional plan and decisions concerning management of behavior problems. Although most facilities ask families to participate in the planning, if you are not invited to join, tell the director that you want to be a part of the process. Your firsthand knowledge of your relative's likes and dislikes, medical problems and favorite activities or hobbies is helpful to the staff. You can often unravel mysterious behaviors or explain what he or she is trying to communicate.

You should participate in formation of all care plans—in choosing activities and social events, and in overseeing nutrition.

The facility should provide family services that will help you form a satisfactory partnership with the staff and come to terms with the changing situation. The services should include support groups, family counseling, and plenty of scheduled activities that allow families to socialize with their loved one.

In making a comfortable transition from primary caregiver, one of the most important things for families to realize — and accept — is that the staff will not always be able to do things exactly the way you did them at home. It is best not to have an antagonistic relationship with the staff. They are trained professionals and develop close emotional ties to the residents. It's important that you trust them, and that they are able to do their jobs without your constant worry or criticism.

Establishing a warm, cooperative relationship with the staff helps your family member. If you run into any problems with care, you will be able to discuss them more constructively. However, if you do have a genuine conflict with a staff member or valid objections on how care is being provided, don't argue about it — take steps:

- Contact the director to make your concerns known.

- Ask for a care team meeting so all staff members can work with you to find solutions.

- Bring in an outside professional as a consultant — a doctor, social worker or psychiatrist who specializes in Alzheimer's.

- Increase the number of days a week you visit. For example, if you feel that meal times are not being handled correctly, you can be there to help feed your loved one. But don't take over. What you want to do is change how the staff provides care. That means they must stay involved.

- Ombudsmen are available in every county to mediate or investigate when a conflict can't be managed by the methods above.

SCHEDULING VISITS

Care facilities should welcome family visits at any time without notice, but it may be in the best interest of your loved one to establish a sched- 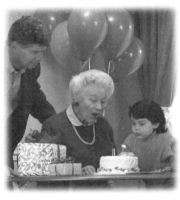 ule. The travel time to the facility, your work and home schedule and your loved one's response to visitors all affect the frequency. Some people choose to make brief visits every day, others find three times a week or once or twice on weekends is the right choice. You'll have to experiment to see what is best for your relative and for you.

Arranging for regular participation in the facility's social events is also a good idea. Group outings, picnics, weekly arts or crafts projects and holiday celebrations can bring a great deal of pleasure to both the family and the person with Alzheimer's.

If you are not going to be able to make a regularly scheduled visit, notify the staff ahead of time so they can prepare your family member for the change, if necessary.

LEARNING HOW TO INTERACT WITH YOUR LOVED ONE IN THE NEW ENVIRONMENT

When you begin visiting your loved one in his or her new home, you will have to learn how best to insert yourself into his or her ongoing life. When you arrive, your relative may be involved in a group activity or may be in an unreceptive mood. You may want all his or her attention, but it may not be appropriate or possible. Each visit may be different.

Flexibility is the key to making your visits go well. If you arrive with a set agenda or rigid expectations, you may feel disappointed or rejected. Go with the flow.

Some days you may simply observe, and sometimes you'll join in group activities. Other times you can spend time together—styling his or her hair, helping with getting dressed, sharing a meal or talking.

Try not to react negatively if your relative doesn't recognize you or understand that you are a special person in his or her life. Even in the more advanced stages of the disease, the person responds to the feelings of affection and love. He or she may not identify the source, but being in the presence of someone who cares improves the quality of life. "When I would visit my husband," recalls a woman whose spouse no longer recognized her, "he would often spend time holding hands with another resident. But I knew he thought he was with me. I felt the love we had shared, even if he couldn't express it directly to me."

How to Handle...

AN UPSETTING VISIT

Sometimes visiting your loved one will fill you with sorrow or bittersweet emotions. He or she may be severely agitated or seem lost in space. You long for connection, but it is elusive. As you return home, you may feel the sharp sting of life's cruelty.

Nothing can prevent these moments. Watching your loved one drift away is painful, sometimes unbearably so. But for your health and for the well-being of your loved one you want to find ways of coping with these emotions.

- Most important, don't deny them.
- Don't bottle them up. Talk to friends, family, social workers. Go to a support group. Make yourself open to the help and insights of others.
- Remember the good times. You have many precious memories. Your life together is not confined to the present difficulties but has blossomed over the years. And those years created wonderful, shared experiences that are still part of your life — and of your loved one's. They should not be erased by the current hardships.
- Find solace and humor in who the person is today. Focus on the strengths and positives of the situation instead of the deterioration.
- Develop new creative ways of enjoying your time together. Try looking at old pictures together, reminiscing, watching TV, sitting quietly, taking a walk, joining up with another resident and his or her visitors.
- Go visit again soon. Don't deny yourself a pleasurable visit because of a painful one. Each visit is different — both you and your loved one will be in a different mood the next time you see one another.

My Grandfather's Gift

BY ALAN THICKE

*Actor Alan Thicke found sadness mingled
with profound appreciation
as he watched his beloved grandfather pass through
the stages of progressive dementia.*

"My grandfather Willis and I were very close. My parents were divorced when I was six and I lived with my grandparents. Even after my mother remarried, I'd spend summers with them.

"They lived in Kirkland, Ontario. It's a 12-hour trip from Los Angeles, but I'd take my kids up on a little single engine plane, landing on frozen lakes, to visit him. He was so dear, it was important that my kids know who he was and be in touch. They were very fond of him.

"When he and his wife could no longer care for themselves — he developed dementia and she was not strong enough to handle everything — they moved together into a local nursing home. It was hard for her. She was in denial and would get mad at him if he couldn't remember her name. But even when he was no longer coherent, he gave me and my children a feeling of family and taught us the power of family love. He made us realize that love is not contingent upon how the outer person functions. It grows from an inner well of feelings and shared concern. That was his gift and every day I treasure the memory.

"I would say to other families, if your loved one is not in any mental or physical pain, then just cross your fingers and enjoy whatever fragments are left. Identify what you can still relate to that will be meaningful to both of you. Nourish whatever cells are left to 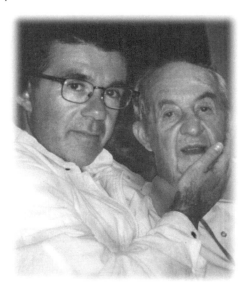 challenge. That enjoyment is important not only for your loved one but for the family. If you agonize and moan over the situation, then that's only further damaging to the family.

"When we'd go up and visit him at the nursing home, there was no sense in telling him in advance. We'd simply get off the elevator and he'd be sitting there looking into space. But when we'd wave and call his name, something would come over his face.

"Towards the end he couldn't have sensible conversations, but he knew that a loved one was there for him. I think he lived in a benign confusion and that allowed us to keep a sense of humor about it all.

"He'd do amusing things. His old job was as a car sales-man and occasionally he would try to sell us a car. And once he had the kids and me all waiting for King George to come over and play hockey. Spending time with him consisted of looking for fragments of sentences and feeding him and just being there for him. Of course there was sadness, but we would have been delighted to have a couple more years of him shuffling along the hall. We were phased out of his life and his consciousness over the course of a year and a half.

"Willis was 82 when he died of pneumonia. Until the end, he was an important person to his wife and to me and my children. He gave us all a feeling of love and family."

Appendix

Agency for Health Care Policy & Research
(AHCPR) Clearinghouse

(an arm of the U.S. Department of Health and Human
Services)

P.O. Box 8547

Silver Spring, MD 20907-8547

Phone: 800-358-9295

Screening for Alzheimer's Disease is due out in 1996.
Call the toll-free number to order your copy.

Alzheimer's Association

National Headquarters

919 North Michigan Ave.

Suite 1000

Chicago, IL 60611-1676

Phone: 800-272-3900

This is the largest national, nonprofit volunteer group dedicated to Alzheimer's research and education. There are more
than 200 chapters and 2,000 support groups across 50
states. Check local phone directory for chapters, or call
800-272-3900. They offer a free quarterly Alzheimer's
Association newsletter, along with numerous publications,
including: *Family Guide for Alzheimer's Care in Residential*

Settings; *Steps to Home Care*; *Steps for Selecting Activities*; *Steps to Choosing a Physician*; *Just the Facts and More* (package/fact sheets); and *Guidelines for Dignity: Goals of Specialized Alzheimer's/Dementia Care in Residential Settings*, which outlines key components of nursing homes and other facilities that care for people with memory impairments.

The *Safe Return* program is a nationwide registration and bracelet identification program for those with memory loss.

Alzheimer's Association Public Policy Office

1319 F St., NW, Suite 710

Washington, DC 20004

Phone: 202-393-7737

Alzheimer's Association 1995 Advocate's Guide to National Policy Priorities outlines key federal and state public policy issues, referencing specific legislation and suggesting advocacy action steps; *Long-Term Care: The Hidden Healthcare Crisis in Rural America* presents new census data on long-term care problems in rural states; *Alzheimer's Advocate Handbook*, an easy-to-use guide for the individual advocate, offers tips in letter writing, meeting with public officials and getting results; *State Policy Report* is a free, bimonthly newsletter highlighting key legislative and regulatory developments of interest to Alzheimer's advocates.

Alzheimer's Disease Education & Referral Center (ADEAR Center)

(Sponsored by the National Institute on Aging)

P.O. Box 8250

Silver Spring, MD 20907-8250

Phone: 800-438-4380

The toll-free number links callers to information specialists who can respond to inquiries from the general public, patients, family members and professionals. In addition, they offer 20 free publications on Alzheimer's disease and related disorders, including an annual progress report on Alzheimer's research and an Alzheimer's disease fact sheet. They can also refer callers to one of the 28 Alzheimer's research centers nationwide (see below) for diagnostic services, offer training materials for caregivers, and help find a doctor in your area.

Alzheimer's Disease Research Centers

The National Institute on Aging has set up 28 Alzheimer's Disease Centers (ADC) at state universities across the country. They offer diagnostic and treatment services, along with information about the disease, services and resources. Volunteers can participate in drug trials and other clinical research projects. Call 800-438-4380 for an ADC Program Directory.

Alzheimer's Foundation

8177 South Harvard St., Suite 114

Tulsa, OK 74137

Phone: 918-481-6031

This is an international organization focused on research and cost-effective caregiving issues.

American Association of Homes and Services for the Aging (AAHSA)

901 E Street NW, Suite 500

Washington, DC 20004-2037

Phone: 202-783-2242

Call for a complete publication list, including *The Nursing Home and You: Partners in Caring for a Relative with Alzheimer's.*

American Association of Retired Persons (AARP)

Fulfillment

601 E Street, NW

Washington, DC 20049

Phone: 202-434-2277

Free single copies available of *Miles Away and Still Caring: A Guide for Long-Distance Caregivers; Staying at Home: A Guide to Long-Term Care and Housing; Medicare: What It Covers, and What it Doesn't;* and *Tomorrow's Choices: Preparing for Future Legal, Financial and Health Care Decisions.*

American Health Assistance Foundation

15825 Shady Grove Road

Rockville, MD 20850

Phone: 800-437-2423

Provides grants to assist in covering the cost of respite care.

American Journal of Alzheimer's Disease

470 Boston Post Rd.

Weston, MA 02193

Phone: 617-899-2702

A journal devoted to issues related to Alzheimer's, including treatment, medical and social research, book reviews, etc. Also available through some public libraries and various branches of the Alzheimer's Association.

Better Directions
Multimedia Products, Inc.

P.O. Box 3064

Waquoit, MA 02536

Phone: 800-999-0795

Publishes *Wiser Now,* a monthly newsletter for Alzheimer's caregivers.

Consumer's Information Center

Dept. 550B

Pueblo, CO 81009

Write for a free 35-page booklet titled: *Alzheimer's Disease.*

Duke University Medical Center
Duke Alzheimer's Family Support Program

P.O. Box 3600

Durham, NC 27710

Phone: 919-660-7510

(Toll-free in North Carolina: 800-672-4213)

The Caregiver newsletter is published three times a year. The Center also publishes manuals, brochures and videotapes for professionals and families. Ask for a publications order form that lists all available materials, including *Sexuality and the Alzheimer's Patient* and *When Your Friend Has Memory Problems: For the Senior Center Participant* (pamphlet).

French Foundation for Alzheimer's Research

11620 Wilshire Blvd., Suite 820

Los Angeles, CA 90025

Phone: 800-477-2243

Twice a year the foundation publishes *High Notes*, a free newsletter on the latest Alzheimer's research.

Johns Hopkins University Press

Hampden Station

Baltimore, MD 21211

Phone: 800-537-5487

Publishers of *The 36-Hour Day*, by N. Mace and P. Rabins.

LRP Publications

747 Dresher Rd., Suite 500

P.O. Box 980

Horsham, PA 19044-0980

Phone: 215-784-0860

Publishers of *Parent Care Advisor*, a monthly newsletter.

ManorCare Health Services

333 N. Summit

Toledo, OH 43604

Phone 800-736-4427

With more than 35 years of experience in the heath care industry, ManorCare Health Services is one of the nation's leading providers of Alzheimer's services and skilled nursing, rehabilitation and assisted living care. They own and operate nearly 200 facilities in 28 states. One of their primary goals is to help educate consumers – through quarterly caregiver newsletters, caregiving seminars, videotapes and informational brochures – so they can make informed choices about caring for their family members.

For more information on care options or to obtain free literature on their public service programs, call the number above.

National Institute on Aging Clearinghouse

P.O. Box 8057

Gaithersburg, MD 20898-8057

Phone: 800-222-2225

The Clearinghouses's free Caregiving Packet contains three pamphlets: *Finding Good Medical Care, Getting Your Affairs in Order* and *When You Need a Nursing Home.* It also contains a guidepost copy of *Aging Parents,* which includes a list of references for the caregiver.

National Institute on Mental Health (NIMH)

Office of Scientific Information (OSI)

Information Resources and Inquiries Branch (IRIB)

5600 Fishers Lane/Room 7C-02

Rockville, MD 20857

Phone: 301-443-4513

NIMH specializes in research on mental illness and the brain. Their free 40-page booklet, *Alzheimer's Disease*, contains information on the latest research in the diagnosis and treatment of Alzheimer's, along with a list of other information resources. To receive this booklet, or other related publications, via fax, call their Mental Health FAX4U line at 301-443-5158. You can also call or write for information.

National Institute on Neurological
Disorders and Stroke

NIH

P.O. Box 5801

Bethesda, MD 20824

The Institute's primary function is to provide federal funding for Alzheimer's research. Send a written request for an information packet on Alzheimer's disease and research.

National Mental Health Services Knowledge
and Exchange Network

P.O. Box 42490

Washington, DC 20015

Phone: 800-789-2647

Call to request free publications and resources on Alzheimer's disease and caregiving, or to order NIMH's updated *Mental Health Directory 1995,* which lists state and city organization associations for residential and partial-care services, and national mental health organizations and related resources. The network also makes referrals to associations.

New York State Office for the Aging

2 Empire State Plaza

Albany, NY 12223-1251

Phone: 518-474-5731; or 800-342-9871 (NY State only).

Call or write for a free copy of *Teenager's Guide to Caregiving.*

Terra Nova Films

9848 South Winchester Ave.

Chicago, IL 60643

Phone: 312-881-8491

This group specializes in films on aging. They've recently produced the award-winning videotape, *A Thousand Tomorrows: Intimacy and Sexuality in Alzheimer's Disease.*

United Seniors Health Cooperative

1331 H St., NW, Suite 500

Washington, DC 20005

Phone: 202-393-6222

A membership organization, the cooperative specializes in insurance counseling. Call to request a free catalog of publications, including: *Long-Term Care: Dollars and Cents Guide* and *Home Care for Older People: A Consumer's Guide.*

Carol Simpson has been helping families and caregivers deal with Alzheimer's disease since 1987. For eight years, she served as the Executive Director of the Alzheimer's Association of Greater Washington. She is currently the Public Information Manager for Alzheimer's Services for ManorCare Health Services in Gaithersburg, Maryland.

The advice in *At the Heart of Alzheimer's* is a suggestion to caregivers rather than a medical or therapeutic prescription to be used without adaptation to the reader's situation. The author intends to provide readers with a greater awareness of Alzheimer's, and ways they can cope with a loved one stricken with the disease. Few cases of this disease are identical, and readers should always discuss their approach to Alzheimer's with physicians and/or other professional practitioners.

This book has been published as a public service by ManorCare Health Services, Gaithersburg, Maryland.